PROGRESS IN
HAEMATOLOGY: 1

PROGRESS IN HAEMATOLOGY: 1

Edited by

Christopher D. R. Dunn
DSc PhD BPharm (Hons) MRPharmS CBiol FIBiol FRSH

and

Christopher J. Pallister
MSc PhD FIBMS CBiol MIBiol CHSM

© 1998
Greenwich Medical Media Ltd.
219 The Linen Hall
162-168 Regent Street
London
W1R 5TB

ISBN 1 900151 448

First Published 1998

A catalogue record for this book is available from the British Library

Distributed worldwide by
Oxford University Press

Project Manager
Gavin Smith

Production and Design by
Saxon Graphics Limited, Derby

Printed in Great Britain by
Ashford Colour Press Ltd

CONTENTS

Contributors vii

Preface ix

1. **STEM CELL TRANSPLANTATION** 1
    J. M. Bird and D. I. Marks

2. **WHITHER LEUKAEMIA CLASSIFICATION?** 17
    M. Reid

3. **FLOW CYTOMETRY IN HAEMATOLOGY** 35
    M. Macey

4. **DETECTION AND ASSAY OF CYTOKINES:
    AN OVERVIEW** 63
    M. Wadhwa and R. Thorpe

5. **GROWTH FACTORS AND THEIR RECEPTORS
    IN HAEMOPOIESIS** 87
    C. J. Pallister and S. A. Marriott

6. **DIFFERENTIATION AND DEVELOPMENT OF
    B AND T CELLS** 103
    L. S. English

7. **PRODUCTION OF RECOMBINANT
    ERYTHROPOIETIN: A BRIEF HISTORY** 135
    C. D. R. Dunn and S. A. Marriott

8. **NADPH OXIDASE: ITS STRUCTURE AND ROLE** 155
    J. T. Hancock, P. J. Moulton and R. Desikan

Index 173

CONTRIBUTORS

David I. Marks and **Jennifer M. Bird**
Bone Marrow Transplant Unit, Bristol Children's Hospital,
St Michael's Hill, Bristol BS2 8BJ, UK

Mike Reid
Royal Victoria Infirmary,
Queen Victoria Road, Newcastle upon Tyne NE1 4LP, UK

Marion Macey
Department of Haematology, The Royal London Hospital,
Whitechapel, London E1 1BB, UK

Meenu Wadhwa and **Robin Thorpe**
Division of Immunobiology,
National Institute for Biological Standards and Control,
Blanche Lane, South Mimms, Potters Bar EN6 3QG, UK

Christopher J. Pallister and **Shirley A. Marriott**
Department of Biological and Biomedical Sciences,
University of the West of England at Bristol,
Coldharbour Lane, Bristol BS16 1QY, UK

Leonard S. English
Department of Biological and Biomedical Sciences,
University of the West of England at Bristol,
Coldharbour Lane, Bristol BS16 1QY, UK

Christopher D. R. Dunn and **Shirley A. Marriott**
Department of Biological and Biomedical Sciences,
University of the West of England at Bristol,
Coldharbour Lane, Bristol BS16 1QY, UK

John T. Hancock, Paul J. Moulton and **Radhika Desikan**
Department of Biological and Biomedical Sciences,
University of the West of England at Bristol,
Coldharbour Lane, Bristol BS16 1QY, UK

PREFACE

Haematology is a rapidly moving subject. Facilitated by the relative ease by which tissue can be obtained, the study of blood and the blood-forming organs is an established research area in its own rights as well as serving as a 'test bed' for various other mammalian tissues. Against this background, teaching haematology to students of medicine, veterinary medicine or the biomedical sciences is especially difficult as the rapidity of change makes everyone uncertain about what is today's version of 'correct', and how tomorrow's data may modify that conclusion. Conventionally, the way to keep abreast of the latest developments is through original, peer-reviewed papers, but these are often very complex and too narrowly focused to meet the needs of all but the most persistent of students.

This book – the first in a series – is intended for the majority of students who need something in the way of a 'bridge' between their current level of knowledge and that expected of readers of original articles. The articles are intended to help students interpret the latest findings in haematology, to provide a backdrop for future advances; and to stimulate more focused and in-depth reading for those wishing to follow a laboratory- or clinically-based career. As such, it is aimed primarily at final-year undergraduate students, and those embarking on studies for a post graduate qualification.

Each of the eight contributions is written by experts in the relevant fields and is intended to be 'information rich' rather than 'reference rich'. Thus, bibliographies are strictly limited to a few, generally recent, references which provide signposts for further reading. Subject-matters have been selected to cover particularly fast moving areas. e.g. stem cell transplantation, FACS, cytokines and NADPH oxidase, as well as those in which some time for careful evaluation might be prudent given the rapid advances of the past few years. e.g. erythropoietin. Some of the subjects covered perhaps fall into areas that seem particular adept at assimilating new data and reinterpreting old, e.g. leukaemia classification and lymphocyte development. Each contribution follows a similar overall format of an introduction written at least partly from an historical perspective; an overview of the most recent findings and how they fit with the more established views; and a brief conclusion in which possible fruitful future lines of research are identified.

The chapters therefore provide resumés of the latest advances in the subjects; are intended to go one step further than final-year undergraduate lectures; and for students contemplating a career in haematology to serve as a focus for further reading and for topics most likely to be particularly interesting and rewarding in the future. Subsequent editions in this series will include chapters on such diverse subjects as blood banking, haemoglobinopathies, folate metabolism, cell adhesion molecules, thrombophilia and oncogenes in haematology.

Christopher D. R. Dunn and Christopher. J. Pallister
December 1997

1

STEM CELL TRANSPLANTATION

J. M. Bird and D. I. Marks

SUMMARY

The aim is to provide an understanding of the biology of stem cell transplantation (SCT), the complications that are to be expected and the results that can be achieved rather than a detailed review of all aspects. The paper concludes with some speculation about future developments and the refinements that can be expected of what is now a fairly non-specific tool.

INTRODUCTION

Stem cell transplantation (SCT) refers to the intravenous administration of haematopoietic stem cells to patients to restore normal function to damaged or diseased bone marrow. Stem cells can be derived from the patient (autologous SCT); an HLA-matched or partially matched sibling or unrelated donor (allogeneic SCT); or, less commonly, from an identical twin (syngeneic SCT).

A BRIEF HISTORY

There have been a number of scientific landmarks in the development of SCT. In 1949, Jacobson and colleagues were the first to show that shielding of haematopoietic tissue could alleviate the myelosuppressive effects of total body irradiation. Later work in the 1950s by Ford and Nowell showed that the protection afforded by SCT was due to a transfer of living cells and the induction of immunological tolerance. Barnes, in 1956, proposed that allogeneic SCT had a curative effect not solely due to the tumour cell killing mediated by chemoradiotherapy, and, in 1965, Mathé used the term 'adoptive immunotherapy' for the antitumour effect of allogeneic stem cells. Van Bekkum showed in 1956 that intravenous infusion of marrow after myeloablative treatment could repopulate the marrow space, and in 1967 that marrow could mount an immune response against the host – a condition known as graft versus host disease (GVHD).

In 1972, Thomas reported the first successful allogeneic transplant for severe aplastic anaemia, and 5 years later the results of the Seattle group's first 100 allografts for end-stage acute leukaemia were presented. Evidence that stem cells could be obtained from peripheral blood was first shown in the dog in 1964. Combined immunosuppression with cyclosporin and methotrexate was shown to be effective in preventing GVHD first in dog and later in man.

Autologous SCT was first used successfully to cure patients with lymphoma in the late 1970s and its use became widespread in the following decade. The annual number of autologous stem cell transplants worldwide now greatly exceeds the number of allogeneic transplants.

RATIONALE FOR STEM CELL TRANSPLANTATION IN MALIGNANT DISEASES

Standard doses of chemotherapy and/or radiotherapy may be insufficient to cure many malignant diseases. The primary rationale for high-dose chemoradiotherapy and SCT is that it provides the opportunity to increase greatly the dose of cytotoxic therapies but avoids the associated severe and often fatal myelotoxicity. A secondary (but sometimes equally important) reason is that allogeneic SCT may provide the recipient with immunologically competent cells capable of recognizing and destroying malignant cells in the host.

SOURCES OF STEM CELLS AND GRAFT PROCESSING

Autologous stem cells reinfused after high dose chemoradiotherapy can be derived from the bone marrow or peripheral blood (or a combination of both).

Following chemotherapy there is a rebound recovery of bone marrow which produces a massive release of stem cells in the circulation. This effect is amplified by the use of growth factors or can be achieved by the use of growth factors alone. Optimization of peripheral blood stem cell (PBSC) mobilization and the development of improved apheresis machines have now reached the level where one leucopheresis procedure is often sufficient to collect adequate PBSC for engraftment following transplantation after high-dose chemoradiotherapy. However, in practical terms, stem cell leucapheresis can involve being connected to a leucapheresis machine for approximately 4 h per day for up to 3 days. A bone marrow harvest can be performed under general or regional anaesthetic; takes 45–90 min; and involves the donation of 800–1500 ml for an adult recipient.

There are several advantages when using peripheral blood over bone marrow as the source of stem cells: PBSC provide more rapid engraftment; their collection does not involve a general anaesthetic; and PBSC can be collected in situations when a bone marrow harvest would be difficult or impossible – for example, when the patient has undergone previous pelvic radiotherapy.

Allogeneic stem cells can also be obtained from either the marrow or peripheral blood, although there may be ethical concerns in giving growth factors to unrelated donors. In addition, stem cells may be qualitatively different when obtained from peripheral blood than from bone marrow. The majority of allogeneic transplants continue to use bone marrow rather than peripheral blood as the source of stem cells. There is increasing interest in the use of cord blood from a related or unrelated donor as the source of stem cells, and frozen cord blood banks have been established for patients who do not have a suitable sibling or unrelated donor.

The minimum number of stem cells needed to achieve prompt engraftment is uncertain but most transplanters aim to give $>2\times10^6$ CD34+ cells/kg. There is now evidence that higher cell counts may be beneficial in unrelated and sibling donor SCT. The 14-day granulocyte-macrophage colony-forming unit assay (CFU-GM) is a widely used measure of reconstitutive capacity, but correlations between this assay and speed of engraftment have not always been good.

ABO-compatible allogeneic marrow is generally infused fresh after bone marrow harvest, but autologous stem cells are usually depleted of erythrocytes, cryopreserved with dimethylsulphoxide, and thawed before reinfusion. Depending on ABO incompatibility, stem cells may need to be depleted of erythrocytes or plasma. T cells, which are major mediators of GVHD, may be removed by a variety of techniques including physical methods such as elutriation and immunological methods such as the use of monoclonal antibodies.

PURGING

In autologous SCT, the infusion of stem cells from the patient can contribute to relapse if the transplant contains residual tumour cells. Purging refers to attempts to manipulate the transplant to reduce the possibility of contamination with malignant cells. Many different purging methods have been investigated and are broadly divisible into those based on 'negative' or 'positive' selection of stem cells.

Purging based on 'negative' selection focuses on the use of monoclonal antibodies or chemicals with some selective toxicity for the malignant cells. However, most methods have an effect on the quantity and quality of cells infused and on the speed of engraftment. For diseases such as leukaemia or lymphoma, stem cells may be incubated with agents such as mafosfamide or 4-hydroperoxycyclophosphamide. In lymphoma, the SCT may be purged with B or T cell monoclonal antibodies to antigens expressed on lymphoma cells. In myelocytic leukaemias, one purging strategy involves the culture of stem cells in flasks prior to reinfusion as evidence suggests that non-malignant cells may have a growth advantage *in vitro*.

Purging based on 'positive selection' of stem cells involves passing the cells intended for transplantation through CD34 columns.

Methods of detecting small amounts of tumour have shown that purging based on 'negative' or 'positive' selection is effective in reducing contamination. However, it has been harder to demonstrate clinical benefit, and few purging methods have been subjected to randomized studies to compare them with high-dose chemotherapy and reinfusion of unmanipulated stem cells.

IMMUNOLOGY AND HISTOCOMPATIBILITY

The human major histocompatibility complex (MHC) is located on chromosome 6 and codes for cell surface glycoproteins called human leucocyte antigens (HLA). The class I region encodes for peptide-presenting cell surface molecules named HLA-A, HLA-B, and HLA-C. These genes are highly polymorphic and occur in multiple allelic forms. The class II genes encode HLA-DR, HLA-DQ, and HLA-DP. The HLA region is inherited as a unit (two haplotypes) but these genes can be separated by genetic recombination during meiotic division in about 1–2% of cases. For a given patient the chance of a sibling being a genotypic match is about 0.25. The frequency for various alleles differs considerably among ethnic groups. Tissue typing is used for the determination of class I and II specificities. Class I molecules are expressed on most somatic cells and can be detected by serological and molecular techniques. DNA typing is performed for class II alleles using the polymerase chain reaction (PCR) to amplify HLA genes and sequence-specific oligonucleotide probes (SSOP) for a specific nucleotide sequence within an allele – a procedure designated PCR-SSOP. Sophisticated molecular typing is required to select unrelated donors for SCT.

T cells originate from marrow stem cells that migrate to the thymus and express receptors which recognize self antigens which are deleted by negative selection. Cells that express receptors capable of recognizing foreign peptide antigens are selected for export to various organs. Immune recognition is via the T cell receptor. CD4+ T cells recognize MHC class II molecules and minor histocompatibility antigens bound to them. CD8+ T cells recognize class I antigens.

T cells that develop in the host thymus after SCT are rendered anergic or are negatively selected by host thymic epithelial cells and macrophages (tolerance). Failure to do this can result in graft failure or chronic GVHD, and disordered thymic function is postulated to be the mechanism of autologous GVHD.

PREPARATIVE REGIMENS

Myeloablative conditioning therapy of the recipient is needed to eradicate malignant cells; to create physical space for donor stem cells to engraft; and, in the case of allogeneic SCT, to provide immunosuppression to prevent rejection. As myelotoxicity is frequently dose-limiting for cytotoxic chemotherapy, the use of stem cell rescue provides the opportunity to escalate substantially the dose and further to reduce the load of malignant cells.

The standard and best evaluated conditioning regimen is cyclophosphamide (CY: 120 mg/kg) and total body irradiation (TBI: at 1200 cGy in six fractions over 3 days). Probably the next most commonly used regimen is a combination of busulphan and cyclophosphamide (in a regimen known as BuCy2) which is the same as Cy/TBI except busulphan (16 mg/kg in 4 days) replaces the TBI. In sibling allografts for chronic myelocytic leukaemia these two regimens appear to be equivalent in terms of disease free survival but BuCy2 is associated with less extramedullary toxicity.

Expected toxicities of the preparative regimens include myelosuppression, nausea and vomiting, alopecia, and mucositis with the latter often necessitating intravenous feeding and diamorphine. Hair grows back at 4–6 months after SCT although sometimes more thinly than previously. Prolonged pancytopenia means that the patient will require platelet and erythrocyte transfusions, and usually intravenous antibiotics for fever and presumed infection. Occasionally, bleeding and infection are severe but they are rarely life-threatening problems. The multifactorial, prolonged immunosuppression increases the chance of severe bacterial, viral and fungal infections which, to some extent, can be prevented by prophylactic antibiotics and intravenous immunoglobulin.

ENGRAFTMENT

By convention, the day of engraftment is the first of 3 consecutive days that the peripheral blood neutrophil count is $\geq 0.5 \times 10^9/l$. However, megakaryocytic engraftment and independence from platelet transfusions are also important and the time taken to achieve independent platelet counts of $20 \times 10^9/l$ and $50 \times 10^9/l$ are measures of the speed of overall engraftment.

The mechanisms by which stem cells find their way to the marrow cavity are uncertain. Stem cells express adhesion molecules that interact with vascular endothelium and marrow stromal cells. Initial engraftment may occur in the spleen causing it to enlarge and the splenomegaly may be a source of diagnostic confusion with the suspicion of a relapse.

Studies of donor/recipient lymphohaematopoietic chimerism can be useful in confirming engraftment or its failure. Primary graft failure is said to occur when the neutrophils never exceed $0.5 \times 10^9/l$. The risk of graft rejection is influenced by many factors including transfusion-induced alloimmunisation of the recipient against the donor; pre- and post-transplant immunosuppression; and T cells in the donor marrow. Viral infections and the drugs used to counter them can also cause pancytopenia and can be a source of diagnostic confusion. Graft failure is often fatal because second transplants also often fail to engraft and the conditioning required is extremely toxic to the patient as is the prolonged period of neutropenia.

COMPLICATIONS

Graft versus host disease

GVHD is a complication that predominently occurs after allogeneic SCT: it was first recognized in mouse infused with allogeneic marrow and who developed diarrhoea, weight loss, skin and liver abnormalities in a syndrome termed 'runt disease'. Immunologically competent cells in the graft can recognize and destroy foreign host tissue by recognizing tissue antigens not present in the donor. The severity of the reaction is proportional to the number of donor T cells infused thus providing the rationale for T-cell depletion as GVHD prophylaxis. Prophylaxis of GVHD can also be accomplished by immunosuppression, intravenous immunoglobulin and by germ-free environments in aplastic anaemia.

By definition, 'acute' GVHD occurs within 100 days of SCT but usually within the first month. The afferent arm of the reaction is the activation of donor T cells by recipient tissues: the efferent arm is when these T cells secrete cytokines, recruit additional cells and induce histocompatibility antigen expression.

Acute GVHD principally affects three organs:

- The skin (in which the epidermis and hair follicles are the main targets) is often the first organ to be affected and the usual manifestation is the development of an itchy or burning erythematous macular or maculopapular rash classically involving the palm, sole, knuckle, and back of neck or upper torso. This rash can extend, become confluent or, in the worst cases, blister. There is considerable variation in presentation and it can resemble a drug eruption or eczema: skin biopsy can be helpful in confirming the diagnosis;

- The gastrointestinal tract (particularly the intestinal crypts) is the next most commonly involved organ. The most frequently reported symptom is diarrhoea, which is often offensive, green and voluminous. This may be associated with abdominal bloating and pain, nausea, vomiting, and post-prandial epigastric discomfort. Biopsy may show apoptosis of crypt endothelial cells and sometimes a lymphocytic infiltrate. Because the preparative regimens can produce similar gastrointestinal damage, biopsy can be difficult to interpret in the first 20 days after transplant;

- The liver is seldom significantly affected until day 30 and hepatic GVHD usually manifests as painless, progressive jaundice. The most common pattern of liver function test abnormality is an obstructive picture with only modest if any elevations of transaminases. Bile ducts are the target: liver biopsy shows oedema and infiltration of ducts with lymphocytes, sometimes with periportal hepatocytic inflammation. At a later stage there is bile duct drop-out (vanishing bile duct syndrome) and marked cholestasis.

Acute GVHD is graded from I to IV. Grade II–IV disease is regarded as 'significant', requiring systemic treatment with steroids and cyclosporin as first line therapy, with antithymocyte globulin and other immunosuppressives being reserved for more refractory cases.

'Chronic' GVHD is similar to an autoimmune disease and may be related to thymic damage (due to acute GVHD or age) and an inability to delete autoreactive cells. Chronic GVHD affects the same organs as acute GVHD and also the lung. Severe involvement of the skin may be associated with scleroderma and contractures. Depigmentation and scarring may cause considerable cosmetic problems. The mouth is often markedly inflamed with ulcers and changes resembling lichen planus. Lip biopsy is often helpful. *Bronchiolitis obliterans*, which may be a manifestation of chronic GVHD, is associated with dyspnoea, wheezing and cough, abnormal pulmonary function tests, repeated chest infections, and pneumothoraces. However, the immune dysregulation of chronic GVHD and its therapy predispose the patient to severe infections that are an important cause of late post-transplant mortality.

IMMUNE RECONSTITUTION AND INFECTION

White blood cells generally reappear in the circulation 12–21 days after transplant. While neutrophils and monocytes are functional, T and B lymphocytes are functionally impaired for a protracted period because of the time required to 'educate' new lymphocytes in a foriegn environment, and because GVHD and immunosuppressive agents cause lymphopenia. B lymphocytes recover in about 3 months but quantitative and qualitative T cell recovery takes longer. IgG and IgM return to normal by about a year but IgA takes longer to recover.

The problem of when to revaccinate after allogeneic transplant is controversial. Killed vaccines may be given at 12–18 months but measles should probably be delayed until 24 months. Response to vaccines may be poor in the presence of GVHD. Passive immune therapy with intravenous immunoglobulin can decrease bacterial infections and GVHD and is routinely used.

INFECTION

There are many reasons for the post-tranplantation increase in susceptibility to infection. Breaches of oral and gut mucosa predispose to infection with mouth and gut organisms. Hickman lines are mainly infected with Gram-positive organisms, such as *Staphylococcus*, particularly *S. epidermidis*, but can be colonized with resistant Gram-negative bacteria or fungi.

Patterns of immune recovery are reflected in the predictable times that infections occur after transplant. In the first 21 days, recipients are susceptible to bacterial infections and, if they are profoundly neutropenic for more than 14 days, are liable to fungal infections. Viral infections (e.g. cytomegalovirus) are seen 1–2 months after transplantation, and protozoal infections occur mainly in the first year. The commonest cause of late infections is *Pneumococcus* especially in functionally hyposplenic patients with chronic GVHD. Late infections are particularly seen in recipients of unrelated donor marrow transplants. *Herpes simplex* is mainly seen in the first 5 weeks post-tranplant but *H. zoster* can occur after more than a year. Fungal infections with *Candida* or *Aspergillus* occur in patients with prolonged neutropenia (or graft failure) or exposure to steroids for GVHD. The role of gran-ulocyte transfusions is much debated but they may have a role to play in patients with severe neutropenia and refractory life-threatening infection.

SOME LONG-TERM COMPLICATIONS

In children, growth and development may be compromised by SCT. Several fac-tors influence the incidence of these problems including prior chemotherapy or radiotherapy, the conditioning regimen (whether or not TBI is used), allogeneic or autologous SCT, post-SCT therapy (particularly steroid treatment), and final-ly the presence of chronic GVHD. Growth may be affected in several ways:

- growth hormone deficiency resulting in poor growth and inadequate pubertal growth spurt;

- defects of spinal growth resulting in skeletal disproportion;

- local growth defects particularly of the hair, teeth and facial bone;

- thyroid dysfunction (see below); and

- delayed puberty and gonadal dysfunction.

Secondary malignancies occur after transplant at a significantly higher frequency than in a control population. Data from the International Bone Marrow Transplant Registry (IBMTR) suggests an incidence of secondary malignancies of about 0.6 per 100 patient years in transplant recipients and most are fatal. These tumours include EBV-associated lymphoproliferative disease and donor cell leukaemias. TBI appears to be a risk factor, as does the use of antithymocyte glob-ulin to treat GVHD.

Overt hypothyroidism occurs in about 10% of patients after TBI although fraction-ating the dose may reduce the risk. Treatment is with thyroxine. Thyroid tumours may also be more common in transplant recipients than in the general population.

Cataracts are seen in about 50% of patients who receive 12 Gy fractionated TBI, with the risk seemingly lower in chemotherapy-conditioned patients (about 20%). Implantation of an artificial lens is the treatment.

INDICATIONS FOR SCT

Controversy surrounds many of the conditions for which SCT is sometimes used. However, there is good evidence the procedure is beneficial for:

- HLA-matched sibling allografts in:
  (1) chronic myelocytic leukaemia in first chronic phase;
  (2) standard or poor risk acute myelocytic leukaemia in first complete remission;
  (3) acute lymphocytic or acute myelocytic leukaemia in second complete remission and Philadelphia-positive acute lymphocytic leukaemia in first complete remission;
  (4) very severe aplastic anaemia;
  (5) the myelodysplastic syndromes refractory anaemia with excess blasts (RAEB) and refractory anaemia with excess blasts in transformation (RAEBt); and
  (6) young patients with multiple myeloma in complete remission or near-complete remission.

- Similarly, well-matched unrelated donor transplants are accepted therapy in:
  (1) young patients with chronic myelocytic leukaemia in first chronic phase who have failed to respond to interferon;
  (2) Philadelphia-positive acute lymphocytic leukaemia; and
  (3) young patients with severe myelodysplastic syndromes.

- Autologous stem cell transplants and high dose chemotherapy in:
  (1) chemoresponsive-relapsed intermediate and high-grade non-Hodgkins lymphoma; and
  (2) multiple myeloma for which SCT is superior to chemotherapy but is not curative.

More controversial indications include autografting for high risk stage II breast cancer, acute myelocytic leukaemia in first complete remission, and relapsed germ cell tumours.

No proven role for autografting has been demonstrated for acute lymphocytic leukaemia in second remission, metastatic breast cancer, chronic myelocytic leukaemia and ovarian cancer, or for allografting for standard risk acute lymphocytic leukaemia in first complete remission.

The decision about whether to transplant depends on many factors including:

- the chance of cure with transplant;

- the chance of cure with the alternative therapies;

- expected transplant-related mortality; and
- patient preference.

GRAFT VERSUS TUMOUR EFFECT

There are multiple, well-accepted lines of evidence that the allograft itself contributes to tumour cell kill and cure of the patient. Although the importance of a graft versus tumour (GVT) effect seems to depend on the disease being treated, the evidence in favour of a clinical benefit includes:

- relapse is less common when there is significant acute and chronic GVHD;
- donor leucocyte infusions mediate a clear GVT effect;
- in relapsed disease, withdrawal of immunosuppression may be associated with disease regression; and
- relapse of leukaemia is more common in syngeneic than allogeneic SCT.

There have been many attempts to enhance the GVT effect by:

- reduction of post-BMT immunosuppression;
- use of IL-2 post transplant in patients at high risk of relapse; and
- post-transplant interferon for chronic myelocytic leukaemia and multiple myeloma.

In some animal systems, GVHD can be differentiated from GVT and it is postulated that different effector cells may be responsible. Both CD4+ and CD8+ T cells are involved in GVT, but CD8+ cells seem to be the major mediator. The targets may include MHC antigens on leukaemia cells or leukaemia specific antigens such as BCR-ABL fusion proteins that may be expressed on the cell surface.

DISEASE RELAPSE

Recurrence of disease after achieving a complete remission – relapse – is the most common cause of treatment failure following SCT. It may represent a failure to eradicate sufficient clonogenic malignant cells in the host or, in the case of autologous SCT, reinfusion of malignant cells. It can occur at any time but is most common in the first 3 years after transplant. It usually presents with clinical features similar to those present at diagnosis, e.g. bleeding, infection or anaemia if it is relapsed leukaemia. Anaemia and thrombocytopenia are commonly present as are blasts. A bone marrow biopsy is often necessary to confirm relapse.

The chance of relapse depends on many factors including the stage of disease at transplant, the source of stem cells, the conditioning regimen and the severity of GVHD. Viral infections and graft failure can also cause pancytopenia post-transplantation, and it is important to distinguish relapse from secondary malignancies such as EBV-associated lymphoproliferative diseases. There are also well-documented instances of leukaemia arising from the donor stem cells.

Most diseases that relapse post-SCT are incurable and the choice of therapy is limited to three general types: chemotherapy, immunotherapy and a second SCT. Intensive chemotherapy is often unsuccessful and is poorly tolerated with marked toxicity and prolonged marrow aplasia. This type of therapy is probably only worthwhile if there is a possibility of potentially curative therapy such as donor leucocyte infusion (DLI) or a second SCT. DLI, a form of adoptive immunotherapy, can achieve complete cytogenetic (and often molecular) remissions in >70% of patients with relapsed chronic-phase chronic myelocytic leukaemia, and some of these remissions have lasted >8 years. The results in acute leukaemia are poor, partly because of the pace of the disease and partly becuase the leukaemic cells do not seem as susceptible to a GVT effect. DLI are associated with significant toxicity including GVHD and marrow aplasia, and patients need to be carefully observed.

A second SCT can be curative but is often very toxic because of an increased incidence of veno-occlusive disease, interstitial pneumonitis and infection. However, it can be a feasible procedure when the relapse is >2 years from the first SCT. Considerable thought needs to be given to the conditioning regimen to limit cumulative toxicity and to swing any possible GVT effect in the patient's favour.

THE FUTURE

SCT is a 'sledgehammer' and it is tempting to speculate that, eventually, as the causes of diseases are better understood, the 'sledgehammer' can be dispensed with in favour of far more specific therapies. This may happen some time in the twenty first century, but it would seem likely that we shall have to resort to SCT for some time to come.

Graft engineering

All aspects of SCT are likely to improve, and many of its problems would not exist if there was a clean source of large numbers of pluripotential, self-renewing stem cells. Identification, separation and culture of these cells would eliminate the problem of giving the recipient the malignant cells capable of causing relapse. But stem cells alone will not suffice as a graft. Cells are needed that are capable of mounting an immune response against the tumour being treated, preferably without causing GVHD. These cells may need others to help them function fully in tumour destruction. Yet other cells may be needed to ensure rapid and full engraftment. This concept of graft engineering may allow the cellular components of a graft to be precisely determined in the forseeable future.

Unrelated donors

The use of unrelated donors is likely to increase. Better tissue typing with molecular characterization of class I and II antigens and an understanding of minor antigens will be important. Functional assays that reliably predict the relevance of antigenic differences between donor and host may aid donor selection, and it is possible that some mismatches may become less important in terms of causing rejection or GVHD.

Umbilical cord blood

Human umbilical cord blood is likely to become a more commonly used source of stem cells than at present. Data suggest that the quality and quantity of so-called LTCIC (long-term culture-initiating cells) from umbilical cord blood may be greater than in the marrow or peripheral blood, and that a smaller number of mononuclear cells may be needed to produce durable engraftment. However, to become a practical option, cord blood must be sufficient to engraft an adult, and at the present time clinical and laboratory immunological data are less well understood than with the more widely used sources of stem cells. Claims that a greater degree of mismatch can be tolerated with umbilical cord blood require substantiation by carefully controlled studies. The question of whether cord blood exerts a sufficient GVT effect is also unanswered. There is a worryingly high incidence of failed engraftment with cord blood cells, and at present there is no definite indication for using cord blood when there is a similarly matched unrelated marrow donor.

Ex vivo expansion

Ex vivo progenitor cell expansion is also a very active area of research and there are currently conflicting data about whether it is really possible to expand LTCIC, and not just increase, the number of committed progenitors. A number of investigators have demonstrated >40-fold expansion of these progenitors, but usually at the expense of earlier stem cells. The variety of techniques of assessing stem cell numbers makes it difficult to assess the validity of studies and to compare results. It is possible that the arrival of cytokines such as megakaryocyte growth and differentiation factor and flt-3 ligand may improve results.

Gene therapy

In the future, SCT will increasingly become the vehicle for introducing genes to patients to correct, well-defined, genetically-induced diseases. However, much remains to be done before this becomes an efficient or widely used approach. There has been recent progress in improving the efficiency of retroviral transduction of stem cells, but many other technical problems need to be overcome before gene therapy can be applied to diseases such as β-thalassaemia.

Gene marking of stem cells is being performed in a number of diseases to determine the causes of relapse after autografting.

Infection

Infection is still a major problem and there are no specific therapies for many important viruses. Earlier detection of viral infection by PCR may make existing therapies more effective. Established fungal infections are very hard to cure and early detection by PCR, or prophylaxis in high risk patients, are likely to be the most rewarding strategies. Some late bacterial infection can be prevented by antibiotic prophylaxis but this is not always effective: a better approach may be to prevent the delayed immune reconstitution that underlies the problem.

Patient selection

Finally, one of the most basic problems is which patient to transplant. People are still transplanted whose data suggested that they can be cured by other less drastic means, and SCT is continued in patients who it cannot currently cure but for whom other therapies provide an equally gloomy outlook. Further studies of minimal residual disease may be useful, but the finding of cells with the molecular abnormalities of the original tumour does not guarantee that these cells are clonogenic and capable of causing relapse.

CONCLUSIONS

Stem cell transplantation will become more refined in the future. There will be better sources of stem cells and better prevention and treatment of the complications of transplantation. With an increased understanding of disease processes and more basic knowledge of immunology, we may be able to perform a much more specific and less toxic procedure than we do now.

SELECTED READING FOR MORE DETAILED INFORMATION

This paper showed that SCT could cure a proportion of patients with leukaemia, which could not be treated satisfactorily with any other therapeutic modality:
Thomas ED, Buckner CD, Banaji M *et al*. One hundred patients with acute leukemia treated by chemotherapy, total body irradiation and allogeneic bone marrow transplantation. *Blood* 1977; **49**: 511–533

This is one of the few randomized controlled studies in SCT that show clear benefits for new therapies. It established cyclosporin and methotrexate as standard GVHD prophylaxis:
Storb R, Deeg HJ, Whitehead J *et al.* Methotrexate and cyclosporine compared with cyclosporine alone for prophylaxis of acute graft versus host disease after marrow transplantation for leukemia. *New England Journal of Medicine* 1986; **314**: 729–735

The classic gene marking study that elucidated the origins of relapse after autografting:
Brenner MK, Rill DR, Moen RC *et al.* Gene-marking to trace origin of relapse after autologous bone-marrow transplantation. *Lancet* 1993; **341**: 85–86.

This paper describes and grades post-transplant toxicities:
Bearman SI, Appelbaum FR, Buckner CD et al. Regimen related toxicity in patients undergoing bone marrow transplantation. *Journal of Clinical Oncology* 1988; **6**: 1562–1568

A classic paper describing clinical grading of acute GVHD. Arguably this has left an unwieldy, unreproducible system but it is the system most transplanters use:
Glucksberg H, Storb R, Fefer A et al. Clinical manifestations of graft versus host disease in human recipients of marrow from HLA matched sibling donors. *Transplantation* 1974; **18**: 295–304

A classic paper that classifies and describes chronic GVHD and separates it into limited and extensive groups:
Shulman HM, Sullivan KM, Weiden PL et al. Chronic graft versus host syndrome in man. A long term clinicopathological study of 20 Seattle patients. *American Journal of Medicine* 1980; **69**: 204–217

A landmark paper providing convincing evidence of a GVT effect and the first documentation of curative immunotherapy post-SCT:
Kolb HJ, Mittermuller J, Clemm C et al. Donor leucocyte transfusions for treatment of recurrent chronic myelogenous leukaemia in marrow transplant patients. *Blood* 1990; **76**: 2462–2465

The best all-round textbook of bone marrow transplantation. Good on scientific and clinical aspects, and written by people regarded as the best in their field:
Forman SJ, Blume KG, Thomas ED. Bone marrow transplantation. Boston: Blackwell, 1994

A more clinically oriented book but complementary to the Forman, Blume and Thomas text above:
Atkinson K. Clinical bone marrow transplantation. Cambridge: Cambridge University Press, 1994

A landmark paper in cord blood transplantation:
Wagner JE, Kernan NA, Steinbuch M et al. Allogeneic sibling cord blood transplantation of children with malignant and non-malignant diseases. *Lancet* 1995; **346**: 214–219

A nice review:

Emerson SG. *Ex vivo* expansion of hematopoietic precursors, progenitors and stem cells: the next generation of cellular therapeutics. *Blood* 1996; **87**: 3082–3088

A paper that has changed our thinking about minimal residual disease:

Roberts WM, Estrov Z, Ouspenskaia MV et al. Measurement of residual leukemia during remission in childhood ALL. *New England Journal of Medicine* 1997; **336**: 317–323

2

WHITHER LEUKAEMIA CLASSIFICATION?

M. Reid

SUMMARY

Classification of leukaemia is not simply an academic exercise. It should allow an increase in diagnostic precision and highlight distinct diseases in a superficially homogeneous group, provide clinically and prognostically important information, enable meaningful comparison of different treatments and help improve the understanding of pathogenesis of the disease as well as the normal physiology of a tissue. This review covers morphological, immunophenotypic, cytogenetic, molecular and other classification systems of acute and chronic leukaemias, it highlights new information that in the future may be incorporated into or even replace some already established systems, and stresses the need for adaptability in the construction and reassessment of their worth.

INTRODUCTION

It is useful to know whence one has come when asking whither one might go! The classification of leukaemia is no exception. 'Leukaemia' is a broad church, encompassing a number of acute and chronic disorders – a subdivision which is a classification system in itself but one which will be taken as read. Rather, it is the subclassifications of these disorders that are now of considerable interest and in which change is taking place. This review will consider several broad groups and will not be comprehensive: it will be a brief introduction to current, well-accepted classification systems and will point out areas where progress, modifications and improvement are being made as well as some areas where progress should be made but is being impeded.

One important question should remain at the forefront: what is the purpose of a classification? My view is that its purpose is to:

- increase diagnostic precision and highlight truly different diseases within a superficially homogeneous group;

- provide clinically and prognostically important information;

- enable meaningful comparison of different treatments; and

- facilitate a better understanding of both pathogenesis of disease and of normal physiology of a tissue.

The whole tone of this article reflects my combined interests in laboratory investigation and clinical management. An article written by an immunologist, or other basic scientist, might have had a very different balance.

In approaching this overview I have decided not to include illustrations of typical morphological features. There are numerous excellent atlases of haematology, some even devoted to paediatric haematology, and most haematology departments will have at least one. It would be invidious to suggest a single reference source.

ACUTE LYMPHOBLASTIC LEUKAEMIA (ALL)

Morphological classification

Without going back into the mists of time, the French–American–British (FAB) group's morphological classification is long established and has stood the test of time in at least one respect – the differentiation of L3 ALL from the other two more common types, L1 and L2, remains important and reproducible. Recognition of L3 morphology alerts one to the high probability of B-cell acute leukaemia of Burkitt type. Major differences in therapeutic approach result from such a distinction. The outlook, of children at least, with B cell ALL has been dramatically improved in many countries by treating such cases with aggressive non-Hodgkin's lymphoma therapy. On the other hand, haematologists' ability reliably to distinguish between L1 and L2 ALL remains in some doubt and, in any case, it is only of marginal importance. Few if any changes in therapeutic approach follow from this distinction and differences in outcome are often no longer statistically significant once other prognostic factors have been taken into account.

Immunophenotypic classification

The advent, over the past 25 years, of a wide variety of immunological tests to detect various patterns of expression of cell surface, cytoplasmic and nuclear antigens in leukaemia cells has led to an increase in the knowledge available about the lineage and level of commitment of leukaemia progenitors and to ever more sophisticated models of normal lymphocyte ontogeny (see Chapter 6 by English in this issue). There has undoubtedly been an increase in diagnostic precision but, that apart, it could be argued that an increased understanding of the differentiation of normal T and B lymphocytes has been the main benefit of immunophenotypic investigations of ALL – it has rarely been of much clinical importance to allocate individual cases of ALL to various levels of lymphocyte differentiation/ maturation in whichever model of normal lymphoid ontogeny is in vogue. Currently, most large multicentre trials of ALL recognize null, precursor B (which includes both common and pre-B), B and T ALL.

One very important aspect of immunophenotyping, alluded to above, is the detection of clonal surface immunoglobulin. The consistency with which this has been detected over 25 years, its correlation with L3 morphology and observations of outcome to specific treatment regimens has helped define B ALL in all age groups and now ensures that more appropriate therapy is offered. Our ability to define the category of null ALL (TdT-, CD10-, CD19+) may yet be clinically important. This type of leukaemia occurs more frequently in the infant and adult than in the peak age group of children with ALL, and seems to be associated with a poorer outlook. The value of defining precursor T ALL and distinguishing it from precursor B ALL is somewhat more controversial. Many American studies continue to show an inferior outlook for T ALL. It is not yet clear if subtle but important differences between treatments can explain the variation in outlook.

The clinical importance, and indeed even the reliability of detection, of so-called biphenotypic ALL (expression of myeloid antigens by ALL cells) is also controversial. Such tests are no longer required by current Medical Research Council trials in childhood leukaemia. What were once naively considered 'lineage specific' markers are steadily being realised to be nothing of the sort: one prime example is the frequent expression of CD19, once considered a paradigm of a B-specific marker, by acute myeloid leukaemia blasts in M2 AML.

Possibly the most important immunophenotypic revelation is the relative preponderance of common ALL in Westernized, high socioeconomic-class countries and its relative infrequency in many Third-World countries. This has contributed to considerable speculation and the construction of novel hypotheses about the aetiology of ALL, but it has little relevance to pragmatic clinicians or the management of individual patients.

Cytogenetic classification

A number of important associations between cytogenetic abnormalities and response to treatment have emerged. The Philadelphia (Ph) chromosome, a very small chromosome 22 involved in a reciprocal translocation with chromosome 9 – t(9;22) – was the first cytogenetic abnormality found to be associated with human cancer. (The translocation brings together the *abl* proto-oncogene from chromosome 9 and a region termed the breakpoint cluster region [*bcr*] from chromsome 22. The result of the translocation is a mutant protein – abl-bcr – with enhanced and unregulated tyrosine kinase activity.) It was not long before haematologists realised that the Ph chromosome was not restricted to chronic myeloid leukaemia. It is now known to be present in a small number (perhaps 1–4%) of childhood ALL cases and in many more adults – 13% in young and 26% in older adults in our own regional demographic studies, and accounting for 50% of our older adults with common ALL. It confers an invariably grim outlook in ALL. There is increasing evidence that Ph+ ALL, even that with breakpoints in the minor *bcr* region, is a disease arising out of a pluripotent haemopoietic stem cell, in sharp contrast with models of typical precursor B ALL. This hypothesis has major therapeutic implications whose impact will affect many more adults than children.

Other important translocations include t(8;14) and its rarer variants in B cell (Burkitt's) leukaemia (now excluded from ALL trials, as mentioned earlier), and translocations involving 11q23, which are particularly common in the infant. The 11q23 translocation usually arises in null ALL and also has a very poor outcome with conventional, and even some more aggressive, chemotherapy regimens. One translocation previously associated with poor outcome is the t(1;19), but changes in treatment have resulted in improved survival for these children over the past few years.

Selecting groups with poor outcome has been one traditional occupation for those designing and analysing outcome of large trials. There is some good news, however! High hyperdiploidy (>50 chromosomes per blast) seems to be associated with a better outlook in the child and probably in the young adult too. The drawback of failed cytogenetic analyses has to some extent been countered by measuring the DNA index – approximately the amount of DNA per leukaemia cell divided by the amount per normal cell. Leukaemic patients with a DNA index >1.15 appear to have a very good outcome. Most recently t(12;21), which in most cases is not detectable by classical cytogenetic methods but results in a new hybrid *tel/aml1* gene, has been found to be the single most common genetic rearrangement in childhood cancer, occurring in approximately 30% of childhood ALL cases, and is apparently associated with an outstandingly good outcome. One suspects that most of the patients cured >20 years ago by what would now be considered 'inadequate' treatment had this rearrangement.

Molecular classification

Detailed analysis of immunoglobulin or T cell receptor gene rearrangements has until recently probably been of most value to those who develop models of lymphoid differentiation, maturation and function. However, molecular techniques to reveal important abnormalities such as *bcr/abl* (the molecular hallmark of the Ph chromosome – see above), *mll* gene rearrangements (involved in translocations affecting 11q23) and *tel/aml1* have great potential for identifying cases missed by classical cytogenetic investigations. They are, however, expensive and technically demanding, and may for some time remain outside the routine battery of diagnostic tests. In this area of investigation some degree of centralization of testing, perhaps specifically funded by research or ring-fenced health service funds, is the way forward. As far as clinicians are concerned, the information they provide is little different from cytogenetic studies, but such information could be considered 'harder' data with less need for the sort of time-consuming, labour-intensive subjective interpretation and pattern recognition involved in cytogenetic analysis.

Morphology, immunophentotype, cytogenetics and molecules

Attempts to combine all the data derived from these four classifications into one all-encompassing system have not been successful, probably at least in part because of the potential complexity and enormous number of subcategories which would be created. For many centres treating only modest numbers of patients with ALL there could be as many subgroups as patients! Nevertheless it is clear that highlighting some specific cytogenetic abnormalities is of great potential value. Recognition of the Ph chromosome and 11q23 abnormalities cytogenetically or by molecular genetic methods already influences management of individual patients. If the early observations of the good outcome of patients with *tel/aml1* rearrangements and high DNA index are confirmed in large studies, the whole philosophy of further experimental intensification of treatment in such patients will be in need of a radical rethink. Exciting times lie ahead.

Scoring systems

Gender, age, white blood cell count (and perhaps other factors) seem to be related to outcome, at least in the child. Scoring systems have been devised to help design better therapeutic trials and rationally, albeit empirically, based 'risk directed' therapy. In the UK, for example, the 'hazard score' developed by the Medical Research Council Working Party is important for two reasons: it does seem to pick out a group with a poor outcome, and it is extremely cheap and simple to perform. Management of the child is already being affected by such scoring systems. It remains to be seen whether decisions based on them improve the overall outlook by reducing the number of children destined to do well who might have been subjected to overly aggressive therapy, and by concentrating aggressive or novel therapeutic approaches on those who are expected to fare particularly poorly. Management of the adult with ALL according to perceptions of risk is still in its infancy, not least because of the degree of selection bias in many current randomized trials. It is also likely that modifications of such scoring systems, as with any classification, will become necessary as treatment regimens evolve.

Drug resistance

Attempts to detect intrinsic resistance to one or more of the drugs commonly used to treat ALL are in their infancy, at least in so far as their impact on current treatment is concerned. At present much of the work in ALL has been restricted to small studies of the potential prognostic significance of 'up front' studies of lymphoblast sensitivity to drugs used in initial, remission induction, therapy and to some aspects of thiopurine metabolism. I believe such studies will in due course provide valuable information that will be incorporated in a classification of ALL and will be of practical therapeutic importance. The data may also correlate with some of the biological, but poorly understood, indicators of prognosis mentioned earlier. Some may regard this hope as more a declaration of faith than a realistic assessment of the future.

Now and the future

Table 2.1 shows a brief descriptive outline of the FAB morphological classification of ALL. It should not be used as a substitute for the details presented in the original publication.

Table 2.2 shows one approach to a future meaningful and clinically relevant classification of ALL. I foresee continuing movement in classification of this disease, driven in the main by discovery of those features that can identify subgroups for whom less aggressive therapy may become possible, and for targeting others whose outcome on current therapy remains so grim that entirely novel approaches may be justified. The classification of ALL is set to move from what appears to some as an academic exercise to one of great practical importance. Those who manage childhood ALL are already convinced, but the same is not true for all who look after adult patients. The trick will be to persuade them of the potential importance of some of these specialized investigations. In a worrying number of cases the current feeling is 'why bother?' – a manifestation of concern, if not despair, at the deeply disappointing results of treatment in so many adults with ALL over the past 15 or 20 years.

Table 2.1 – Descriptive outline of FAB classification of acute lymphoid leukaemia (ALL)

Class	Major morphological features
L1	mainly small blasts, little cytoplasm, few nucleoli
L2	larger blasts, more cytoplasm, more prominent nucleoli
L3	often larger blasts, deeply basophilic cytoplasm, prominent vacuolation

Table 2.2 – Clinically important subgroups of acute lymphoid leukaemia (ALL).

Diagnostic tool	Subgroups
Morphology	L3 or not
Immunophenotype	null, common or T
Cytogenetics	Ph – bcr/abl; 11q23 – MLL (poor outlook)
Molecular rearrangement	tel/aml1, DNA index >1.15 (good outlook)
Hazard scores	incorporating gender, age and white blood cell count
Drug resistance	sensitivity to steroids and mercaptopurine metabolism

ACUTE MYELOID LEUKAEMIA (AML)

The FAB group now recognizes eight major subgroups of AML. Essentially a morphological classification, immunophenotypic influences have crept into the definitions of some subtypes, such as M0 AML (blasts should be negative for lymphoid-associated antigens and positive for at least one myeloid antigen) and M7 AML where blasts must express some antigens characteristic of megakaryocytes or contain platelet peroxidase. There are instances of a variant erythroleukaemia where expression of erythrocyte-associated antigens by the blasts may be used to distinguish it from other forms of AML but which, because of the paucity of morphologically identifiable nucleated erythrocytes in the marrow aspirate, would not currently be acceptable as M6 AML. Table 2.3 shows a brief descriptive outline of the FAB classification of AML, without all the details necessary for correct assignment of cases to each category.

The importance of the FAB classification lies in two main areas:

- fundamentally, it has resulted in world-wide acceptance of standard criteria for distinguishing between acute leukaemia and more smouldering forms or preleukaemic conditions, which are generally included in the myelodysplastic syndromes; and

- it has highlighted the close association of M2 AML with the characteristic chromosome abnormality t(8;21), M4 with abnormal eosinophils (M4Eo) with interstitial inversions of chromosome 16 (inv 16), M5 AML with 11q23 abnormalities, especially t(9;11), and M3 AML with t(15;17). In the last case the association between morphology and cytogenetic abnormality is so strong and the morphological features so characteristic that prediction of the cytogenetic abnormality from the

Table 2.3 – Descriptive outline of FAB classification of acute myeloid leukaemia (AML)*.

Class	Major morphological features
M0	AML with minimal differentiation: myeloid antigens, +; lymphoid antigens
M1	AML with little differentiation; >90% blasts
M2	AML with differentiation; <90% blasts, remainder differentiated myeloid series
M3	Promyelocytic leukaemia; abnormal promyelocytes; Auer rods; faggot cells
M4	Myelomonocytic leukaemia (M4Eo, with abnormal eosinophils)
M5	Monoblastic and monocytic leukaemia
M6	Erythroleukaemia; >50% of marrow cells erythroblasts
M7	Megakaryoblastic leukaemia; megakaryocyte antigens; myelofibrosis

* In all cases, blasts constitute >30% of non-erythroid cells in the marrow.

morphology is correct in the majority of cases. This is particularly important because treatment of acute promyeloid leukaemia (M3) now involves the early use of all-*trans*-retinoic acid (ATRA) in most protocols. Molecular detection of genetic rearrangements is steadily growing and the number of well-characterized translocations, such as t(8;21), t(15;17) and others, that can be detected by various molecular biological investigations is rising fast. For clinicians this heralds an era of 'harder' data (as for ALL), which will become increasingly important as 'risk-directed' therapeutic approaches are developed for patients with AML (see below).

Despite the worthy record of achievement of the FAB classification of AML, its proponents and those who use it are aware of increasing numbers of cases that are not adequately covered. It is difficult to confine some individual cases of AML within the constraints of this system. One recent challenging letter amply illustrates the extent of the problem, suggesting a more comprehensive classification comprising 15 different entities. It allows incorporation of immunophenotypic, cytogenetic and molecular details. If nothing else, it is a timely reminder of the morphological and biological heterogeneity of AML. Its complexity and the variety of data that could be obtained for each case of AML immediately raise the spectre of further minor variations from the suggested groups and the possibility of further expansion (fragmentation?) of the classification. There is a need for a system that is flexible enough to accommodate such rare cases without hiding their unusual nature behind a bland front or within an extraordinarily long list of almost unique variants.

The dawn of a prognosis-driven classification has also arrived in AML. Within the 'young' patient with AML (for example, those aged <55 years) some cytogenetic abnormalities are associated with a less grim outlook than others. In some studies, the survival of patients with t(8;21), t(15;17) and inv16 treated with chemotherapy alone approaches that of patients treated with bone marrow transplantation (BMT). In centres with somewhat higher procedural mortality from BMT this has raised a therapeutic dilemma.

Unfortunately for those who would like to see the development of a more clinically relevant, prognosis-driven classification of AML, not only is this disease even more heterogeneous than ALL, but also its incidence increases dramatically with age. For the bulk of patients with this disease (those aged >55 years) there is steadily increasing evidence that it may have evolved from preceding myelodysplasia and be less amenable to current combination chemotherapy schedules. Attempts to demonstrate trilineage dysplasia are, however, often hampered by the paucity of megakaryocytes in diagnostic marrow samples. Considerable refinement of what are at present pretty 'blunt' instruments at detecting such cases is required. Important hurdles to progress over in the diagnosis of this disease are the rarity of AML in the child (whose outlook seems to be better than the adult) and the large number of cases in old patients in many of whom co-morbidity from other causes makes them unsuitable for entry to randomized trials of aggressive treatment. There is thus massive potential selection bias in attempts to improve a prognosis-driven classification of this disease. Age, for whatever combinations of reasons, seems to have a major impact on treatment; the elderly, in general, fare badly indeed.

Finally, at the other extreme of age, it is worth mentioning congenital leukaemia and Down's syndrome. Cases of congenital AML do not necessarily fare badly. Those presenting in neonates and associated with trisomy 21 (whether this is restricted to the AML clone or is a manifestation of Down's syndrome or Down's mosaic) often undergo partial or complete spontaneous remissions, some of which are durable. This transient form of leukaemia may be clinically, morphologically and immunophenotypically indistinguishable from more typical AML in the older child or adult, but its behaviour is exceptional and may involve overexpression of a gene carried by chromosome 21. Quite how trisomy 21 in neonatal AML differs from the apparently identical abnormality in the older patient with AML is unknown. Erythroleukaemia is also over represented in Down's syndrome patients and appears to have an unusually good outcome.

Table 2.4 shows one potential scheme for subdividing *de novo* AML that may be important if 'risk-directed' therapy regimens become available, and which may also be important in the analysis of outcome of current approaches to treatment.

CHRONIC MYELOID LEUKAEMIAS

The chronic myeloid leukaemias comprise a family of leukaemias with overlapping clinical and haematological features. By far the most common is chronic granuloid leukaemia (CGL), associated in >90% of cases with the Ph chromosome. Some important advances have been taken in the morphological classification of these diseases. Galton's earlier work has culminated in the FAB group's morphological classification of chronic myeloid leukaemias showing that, with

Table 2.4 – Potentially clinically important subgroups of acute myeloid leukaemia (AML).

Diagnostic tool	Subgroups
FAB	M0 (distinguish from ALL), M3, M4 Eo, M6 in Down's syndrome
Other morphological	trilineage myelodysplasia especially in the elderly
Cytogenetics	t(8;21) – AML1; t(15;17) – retinoic acid receptor gene
molecular	11q23 – MLL gene, other translocations inv16; trisomy 21 in neonates
Age	>55 years fare badly; congenital leukaemia with trisomy 21

careful morphological examination and differential counts of the peripheral blood, CGL (and Ph positivity and/or *bcr/abl* rearrangement) can be diagnosed with tremendous accuracy, thus reliably differentiating it from atypical CML and chronic myelomonocytic leukaemia (CMML). As with other FAB classifications, haematologists are urged to refer to the original sources rather than relying on a glib précis, for it is in the adherence to detail that such classifications fulfil their promise.

Excessively rare diseases such as juvenile chronic myelomonocytic leukaemia (JCML), infantile monosomy 7 syndrome, and chronic neutrophilic or eosinophilic leukaemias were not considered. In the case of JCML it is relatively easy, in theory, to distinguish it from CGL by morphology, differential counts, cytogenetics and elevated foetal haemoglobin (in JCML), but not necessarily from other types of CMML. However, since JCML has never been seen in the Northern region (and not because we have misdiagnosed it either!) I cannot speak from personal experience.

There remains in some haematologists a reluctance to diagnose CGL in the child, although it is by far the most common myeloproliferative disease even in the child. There is also a regrettable tendency among haematologists and paediatricians to diagnose JCML primarily on the basis of the patient's age. Failure to use diagnostic labels accurately has an insidious and deleterious effect on the ability to think about, investigate and manage these diseases.

I do not foresee major changes in the classification of chronic myeloid leukaemias, at the point of diagnosis, within the near future. However, within CGL, patterns of response to interferon may assume greater importance in tailoring subsequent treatment, particularly when considering the role of BMT in the older patient for whom the morbidity and mortality of transplantation is high.

CHRONIC LYMPHOID LEUKAEMIAS AND LYMPHOPROLIFERATIVE DISEASES

There have been major advances in the classification of these diseases in the past 10 years. A combination of more careful morphological examination of blood smears and the explosion of ever more sophisticated panels of monoclonal antibodies is leading to an increased precision of diagnosis. B cell chronic lymphoid leukaemia (CLL), prolymphoid leukaemia (PLL), hairy cell leukaemia (HCL), splenic lymphoma with villous lymphocytes (SLVL), follicular lymphoma (FL) and mantle cell lymphoma (MCL), as well as other leukaemic T cell proliferations, are now all recognizable disease entities in their own right and can be distinguished one from the other by most laboratories equipped for immunophenotyping.

A few years ago, the FAB group proposed a classification of CLL and related diseases, but increasing availability of antibodies to various CD antigens and experience with their use has already led to some modifications. Scoring systems may help improve the reliability of diagnosis of B CLL and other lymphoproliferative disorders, but have not yet been tested widely or for long enough to be certain.

Cytogenetic abnormalities also play an increasingly important part in the diagnostic classification of lymphoproliferative disorders. Atypical CLL is associated with trisomy 12; MCL with t(11;14); FL with t(14;18); and SLVL with del6q. There is no comprehensive, universally accepted classification of chronic lymphoproliferative disorders that brings together morphology, immunophenotype and cytogenetic investigations. The field is fast moving with developments occurring more rapidly than our ability to test their worth in routine haematological practice.

Haematologists who wish to use panels of monoclonal antibodies to aid diagnosis are advised to consult the original sources. However, Table 2.5 shows a brief scheme for a diagnostic panel that I find useful in my day-to-day laboratory experience and which helps me issue differential diagnoses. I hasten to add that I do not issue opinions without at least a peripheral blood smear to look at. Clinical details, especially from patients outside my own hospital, are sometimes hard to come by!

A variety of clinical staging systems has been developed for B CLL, the most common of all the chronic lymphoproliferative disorders. They are based on a model

Table 2.5 – Useful, every-day panel of immunological investigations of chronic lymphoproliferative disease

	B CLL	B PLL[1]	HCL	HCLv[2]	SLVL	FL	T CLL/ MCL	PLL	LGLL[3]
SmIg	weak	strong	strong	strong	strong	strong	strong	–	–
CD19	+	+	+	+	+	+	+	–	–
CD5	+	–/+	–	–	–/+	+			
CD23	+	–	–	–	–/+	–/+	–/+	–	–
FMC7	V/+	+	+	+	+	+	+	–	–
CD3	–	–	–	–	–	–	–	+	+
CD4	–	–	–	–	–	–	–	–/+	–/+
CD8	–	–	–	–	–	–	–	–/+	–/+
CD16	–	–	–	–	–	–	–	–	+
CD56	–	–	–	–	–	–	–	–	+

[1] Prolymphocytic leukaemia; [2] hairy cell leukaemia variant; [3] large granular lymphocyte leukaemia. HCL is also usually positive for CD11c and CD25; HCL variant for CD11c but not CD25; and SLVL may be positive for either or both.

Table 2.6 – Summary of International Staging System for B-type chronic lymphoid leukaemia (B CLL)

Subtype	Number of involved areas	Haemoglobin (G/dl)	Platelets ($\times 10^9$/l)
A	<3	>10	>100
B	3+	<10	>100
C		<10	<100

of a slowly progressive accumulation of clonal lymphoid cells, and use, as a means of assessing tumour burden, involvement of sites such as cervical, axillary and inguinal nodes, liver and spleen size, and some simple haematological parameters – haemoglobin concentration and platelet count. The International Staging System, a modification of, and which also incorporates, the original Rai system, puts patients in three main groups, A–C. Table 2.6 shows a brief summary of this scheme. Its importance lies in the association between stage and prognosis, and the observation that a good response to initial treatment which results in 'down-staging' (i.e. reduction of the tumour burden) usually confers on the patient the prognosis of the lower stage. The earliest form of CLL, where a modest elevation of the lymphocyte count in peripheral blood (together with bone marrow involvement) is the sole significant abnormality, is associated with long survival; such patients often do not need specific treatment for many years.

There are of course many other factors that have been associated with prognosis. These include the pattern of bone marrow infiltration (diffuse versus nodular), pro-lymphocyte counts, lymphocyte count doubling time, age, sex, karyotype, etc. Few studies have used multivariate regression analysis to determine which are inde-pendent and which dependent prognostic variables, and there are often major prob-lems with selection bias in single-centre and multicentre trials. Very few studies can claim to consist of a near complete census of the incident population of patients with CLL. In practice, once the decision to offer any treatment has been taken, few ther-apeutic decisions are based on such prognostic variables. However, the advent of new drugs, such as fludarabine and cladribine, will require more careful attention to accurate staging so that studies of their role and clinical efficacy can be interpreted.

MYELODYSPLASTIC SYNDROMES (MDS)

Although strictly not leukaemias, some mention of MDS is warranted because many do evolve into AML. Features common to most MDS include peripheral cytope-nias, macrocytosis, dysmyelopoiesis, dyserythropoiesis and abnormal megakary-ocyte morphology. In all cases blasts comprise <30% of non-erythroid cells in the marrow. The FAB group proposed a classification comprising refractory anaemia (RA); refractory anaemia with ring sideroblasts (RARS) – both with <5% blasts in the marrow; refractory anaemia with excess (<20%) blasts (RAEB); refractory anaemia with excess blasts in transformation (RAEBt) in which there may be between 20 and 30% blasts; and CMML. The clinical and haematological overlap between MDS and myeloproliferative disorders or chronic myeloid leukaemias seen in CMML can be confusing but both classifications give enough detail to allow a reasonably secure diagnosis of CMML to be made. In the end, it is irrelevant to pragmatic haematologists which of these larger categories is favoured. There is, of course, considerable room for philosophical differences. Further experience has recognized the existence of hypoplastic MDS, but the difference between this and some forms of hypoplastic anaemia is not always clear in the individual patient.

A wide range of clonal cytogenetic abnormalities is found in MDS. Such abnormalities are particularly useful in helping establish a firm diagnosis, and in distinguishing MDS from reactive dysmyelopoiesis or, in the case of hypoplastic MDS, from classical hypoplastic anaemia. However, apart from monosomy 7, which has gained a reputation for poor outcome in all age groups, the detection of karyotypic evolution over time (associated with impending leukaemic transformation), and the 5q- syndrome (which usually has a long leukaemia-free interval), a clinically useful cytogenetic classification remains more a hope for the future than a current reality. The problem of the multiplicity of cytogenetic abnormalities in MDS is compounded by its increasing frequency in old age. Vigorous investigation of old patients is not common and, as a result, large amounts of data are lacking from those in whom the disease is most frequently encountered.

The importance of the FAB classification in the adult lies in defining groups of patients with differing outlooks. The least likely to transform to AML is RARS, the most likely, RAEBt. Such associations help haematologists plan appropriate therapy for individual patients. In the child, MDS is much rarer and the distinctions are not as useful. However, with some modifications to the basic FAB classification to allow for clinical and cytogenetic data to be included, it is still valuable in helping decide which children may benefit from aggressive therapy. It is also important that children and young adults who receive aggressive therapy are carefully distinguished from those with classical AML so that MDS is not 'hidden' under the general umbrella of AML and potential differences in aetiology, biology and clinical response to treatment forever obscured. Many clinicians, when left to their own devices, have an unfortunate (but sometimes understandable) habit of defining diseases by the treatment regimens employed to treat them and even haematologists are not entirely free of this tendency!

CONCLUSION

Existing leukaemia classifications have much to offer. They already contribute to precision of diagnosis, influence therapeutic decisions and further our attempts to understand biology. For morphological classifications there is no substitute for keeping copies of the original papers beside one's microscope. Classification systems have become most sophisticated in ALL, especially in childhood cases, and are moving most quickly in terms of diagnostic precision in the chronic lymphoproliferative disorders; in the former, definition of potentially clinically meaningful subgroups is outstripping the ability to test their worth. In the latter, the dissection of distinct diseases from a superficially homogeneous group is progressing apace. In general, the widespread investigation of important biological indicators of disease subtypes (cytogenetics, molecular markers, aberrant surface antigen expression, drug resistance, etc.) is still in its infancy and may lead to a proliferation of experimental scoring systems and subclassifications. Not until prospective studies of truly representative groups of patients are carried out will the merits of more sophisticated classifications become clear. But it is already clear that there will be new, important and long-lasting additions to those classifications that already exist. Classifications should remain flexible to remain valuable. It is only when, and if, they become carved in stone that they are doomed to failure and obsolescence.

SELECTED READING FOR MORE DETAILED INFORMATION

These seven papers are the seminal publications from the FAB group and provide the gold standard for morphological classification, with some cytogenetic and immunophenotypic additions. They are essential reading and are also, if kept close at hand, invaluable to practising haematologists:

Bennett JM, Catovsky D, Daniel MT et al. The morphologial classification of acute lymphoblastic leukaemia: concordance among observers and clinical correlations. *British Journal of Haematology* 1981; **47**: 553–561

Bennett JM, Catovsky D, Daniel MT et al. Proposals for the classification of the myelodysplastic syndromes. *British Journal of Haematology* 1982; **51**: 189–199

Bennett JM, Catovsky D, Daniel MT et al. Criteria for the diagnosis of acute leukemia of megakaryocytic lineage (M7). *Annals of Internal Medicine* 1985; **103**: 460–462

Bennett JM, Catovsky D, Daniel MT et al. Proposed revised criteria for the classification of acute myeloid leukemia. *Annals of Internal Medicine* 1985; **103**: 620–625

Bennett JM, Catovsky D, Daniel MT et al. Proposals for the classification of chronic (mature) B and T lymphoid leukaemias. *Journal of Clinical Pathology* 1989; **42**: 567–584

Bennett JM, Catovsky D, Daniel MT et al. Proposal for the recognition of minimally differentiated acute myeloid leukaemia (AML-M0). *British Journal of Haematology* 1991; **78**: 325–329

Bennett JM, Catovsky D, Daniel MT et al. The chronic myeloid leukaemias: guidelines for distinguishing chronic granuloid, atypical chronic myeloid, and chronic myelomoncytic leukaemia. *British Journal of Haematology* 1994; **87**: 746–754

This paper provides a comprehensive review of immunophenotyping and other biological features in childhood ALL. There have been more large-scale and representative studies of immunophenotyping of leukaemia in this field than any other. But continued advances mean that this remains a fluid field:
Pui C-H, Behm FG, Crist WM. Clinical and biological relevance of immunologic marker studies in childhood acute lymphoblastic leukemia. *Blood* 1993; **82**: 343–362

These papers will become landmark publications in correlating biological phenomena with outcome, even though we do not yet understand why or how they affect it:
Trueworthy R, Shuster J, Look T et al. Ploidy of lymphoblasts is the strongest predictor of treatment outcome in B-progenitor cell acute lymphoblastic leukemia of childhood: a Pediatric Oncology Group study. *Journal of Clinical Oncology* 1992; **10**: 606–613

McLean TW, Ringold S, Neuberg D et al. TEL/AML-1 dimerizes and is associated with a favorable outcome in childhood acute lymphoblastic leukemia *Blood* 1996; **88**: 4252–4258

In these papers the range of scoring systems is illustrated and an attempt is made to develop risk-directed therapy:
Mastrangelo R, Poplack DG, Bleyer WA et al. Report and recommendations of the Rome workshop concerning poor-prognosis acute lymphoblastic leukemia in children: biologic bases for staging, stratification, and treatment. *Medical & Pediatric Oncology* 1986; **14**: 191–194

Chessells JM, Richards SM, Bailey CC et al. Gender and treatment outcome in childhood lymphoblastic leukemia: report from the MRC UKALL trials. *British Journal of Haematology* 1995; **89**: 364–372

Smith M, Arthur D, Camitta B et al. Uniform approach to risk classification and treatment assignment for children with acute lymphoblastic leukemia. *Journal of Clinical Oncology* 1996; **14**: 18–24

A tantalizing glimpse of an under-investigated aspect of leukaemia treatment is addressed in these three papers: how do drugs kill, or fail to kill leukaemia cells, and does this have an impact on outcome? Is it possible to detect patients in whom a particular therapeutic approach is probably doomed from the outset?:
Pieters R, Huismans DR, Loonen AH et al. Relation of cellular drug resistance to long-term clinical outcome in childhood acute lymphoblastic leukaemia. *Lancet* 1991; **338**: 399–403

Lilleyman JS, Lennard L. Mercaptopurine metabolism and risk of relapse in childhood lymphoblastic leukaemia. *Lancet* 1994; **343**: 1188–1190

Maung Z T, Reid MM, Matheson E et al. Corticosteroid resistance is increased in lymphoblasts form adults compared with children: preliminary in vitro drug sensitivity adults with acute lymphoblastic leukaemia. *British Journal of Haematology* 1995; **91**: 93–100

Albeit only a letter, this provides a vivid illustration of the potential complexity of an attempt to provide a classification of AML into which all cases might fit:
Eikelboom J, Cull G, Erber W. Time for a new acute myeloid leukaemia classification? *British Journal of Haematology* 1996; **92**: 247–248

This page gives the outcome and other data from the largest demographic study of AML in the elderly:
Taylor PRA, Reid MM, Stark AN et al. De novo acute myeloid leukaemia in patients over 55 years old. A population based study of incidence, treatment and outcome. *Leukemia* 1995; **9**: 231–237

The data in this paper show how the introduction of interferon therapy for CGL can lay the foundation for a valuable, dynamic classification that could alter the treatment options for individual patients:
Allan NC, Richards SM, Shephard M. UK Medical Research Council randomised, multi centre trial of interferon-an1 for chronic myeloid leukaemia: improved survival irrespective of cytogenetic response. *Lancet* 1995; **345**: 1392–1397

This paper contrasts the behaviour of MDS in children with the much more familiar disease in adults, and points the way to important modifications of a classification that originally did not consider children at all:
Passmore SJ, Hann IM, Stiller CA et al. Pediatric myelodysplasia: a study of 68 children and a new prognostic scoring system. *Blood* 1995; **85**: 1742–1750

3

FLOW CYTOMETRY IN HAEMATOLOGY

M. Macey

SUMMARY

Over the past 15 years flow cytometry has developed from a purely research tool to a major adjunct to clinical practice. It is recognized as the principal tool for immunophenotypic analysis of cell types, but it may also be used to measure a variety of cell functions such as metabolic burst activity and phagocytosis. Karotypic analysis for the diagnosis of leukaemias and lymphomas is also feasible, as is the identification of DNA aberrations. These and other applications of flow cytometry in haematology are discussed in this chapter.

HISTORY AND DEVELOPMENT OF FLOW CYTOMETRY

In 1956, Coulter described an instrument in which an electronic measurement for cell counting and sizing was made on cells flowing in a conductive liquid with one cell at a time passing a measuring point. This became the basis of the first viable flow analyser. Later, in 1965, Kamentsky described a two-parameter flow cytometer that measured absorption and back-scattered illumination of unstained cells: it was used to determine cell nucleic acid content and size. This instrument represented the first multiparameter flow cytometer, and the first cell sorter was described that same year by Fulwyler. Use of an electrostatic deflection ink-jet recording technique developed by Sweet, also in 1965, enabled the instrument to sort cells in volume at 1000 cells s^{-1}. By 1967 Van Dilla had exploited the real volume differences of cells to prepare suspensions of highly purified (>95%) suspensions of human granuloctyes and lymphocytes.

However, it is only comparatively recently that advances in technology, including the availability of monoclonal antibodies and powerful but cheap computers, have brought flow cytometry into routine use. Previously, microscope-based static cytometry with cell-by-cell analysis had been the mainstay of most diagnostic work. With the increasing ability to measure up to five parameters on 20,000 cells in 1 s, cell-surface antigen analysis has become almost routine and has not only enhanced the diagnosis and management of various disease states, but also has given new understanding to the pathogenesis of disease.

PRINCIPLES OF FLOW CYTOMETRY

Flow cytometry is a system for sensing cells or particles as they move in a liquid stream through a laser (an acronym for light amplification by stimulated emission of radiation) or light beam through a sensing area where the relative light scattering and colour-discriminated fluorescence of the microscopic particles are measured (Fig. 3.1). Analysis and differentiation of the cells is based on size and granularity, and whether the cell is carrying fluorescent molecules (Fig. 3.2). As the cell passes through the laser beam, light is acattered in all directions and that scattered in the forward direction is proportional to the square of the radius of a sphere and so to the size of the cell or particle. Light may enter the cell and be reflected and refracted by the nuclear contents of the cell, thus the 90° light (right-angled, side) scatter may be considered proportional to the granularity of the cell. The cells may be labelled with fluorochrome-linked antibodies or stained with fluorescent membrane, cytoplasmic or nuclear dyes. Thus differentiation of cell types, the presence of membrane receptors and antigens, membrane potential, pH, enzyme activity and DNA content may be facilitated.

Flow cytometers are multiparameter devices recording several measurements on each cell: therefore it is possible to identify a specific cell population in a heterogeneous population. This is one of the most useful features of flow cytometers, and makes them preferable to other instruments such as spectrofluorimeters, where measurements are based on analysis of the entire population.

Most commercial flow cytometers can make five or more simultaneous measurements on every cell, but some specialized research instruments have considerably greater capacity. A typical flow cytometer consists of three functional units (Fig. 3.1):

- a light source or laser, and a sensing system that comprises the sample/flow chamber and optical assembly;
- a hydraulic system that controls the passage of cells through the sensing system; and
- a computer system that collects data and performs analytical routines on the electrical signals relayed from the sensing system.

Flow cytometers may utilize epifluorescent microscopy or dark-ground laser illumination: in both designs the flow chamber is instrumental in delivering the cells in suspension to the specific point intersected by the illuminating beam and the plane of focus of the optical assembly. Cells suspended in isotonic fluid are transported through the sensing system. Most instruments utilize a lamina/sheath flow technique to confine cells to the centre of the flow stream: this also reduces blockages arising from clumping. Cells enter the chamber under pressure through a small apperture which is surrounded by sheath fluid. This fluid in the sample chamber creates a hydrodynamic focusing effect and draws the sample fluid into

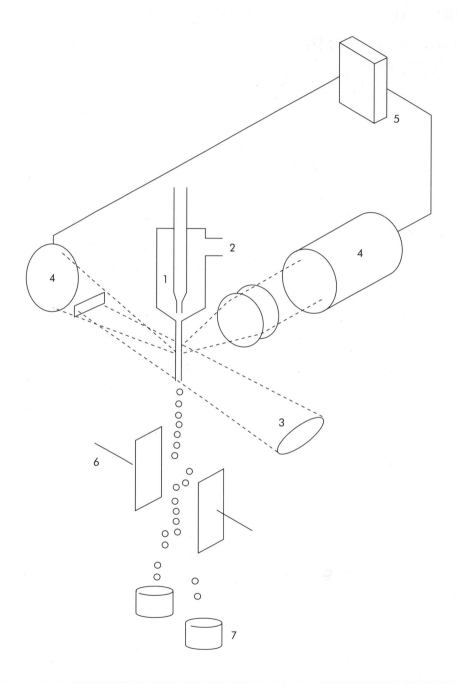

Figure 3.1 – Schematic representation of a flow cytometer. 1, flow cell; 2, sheath stream; 3, laser beam; 4, sensing system; 5, computer; 6, deflection plates; 7, droplet collection.

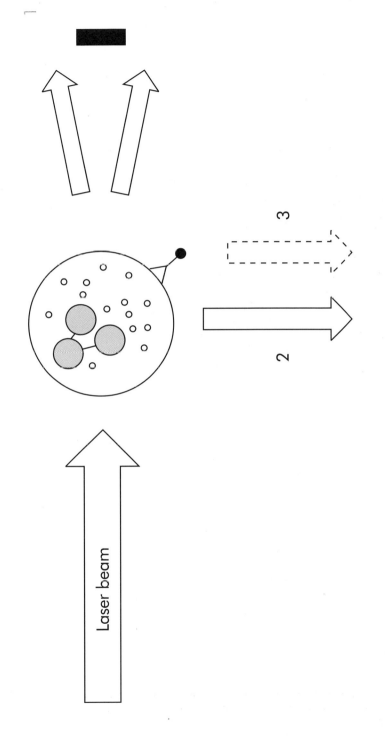

Figure 3.2 – The parameters of flow cytometric analysis. 1, forward angle light scatter; 2, 90°light scatter; 3, fluorescence.

a stream. Accurate and precise positioning of the sample fluid in the sheath fluid is critical to efficient operation of the flow cytometer, and adjustment of the relative sheath and sample pressures ensures that cells pass singly through the detection point. This alignment may be performed manually on some machines, but it is fixed in others.

Chambers used in microscope-based flow systems (where fluorescence is measured in line with the optical system) have limitations. The chamber acts as the horizontal microscope stage, and the top of the chamber is usually a glass coverslip. Scatter measurements are restricted to within the direct optical path of the immersion objectives. Some systems do not use an enclosed channel but simply squirt the hydrodynamically focused sample at a low angle across a microscope slide followed by vacuum aspiration to waste.

In laser-based flow cytometers – where fluorescence is measured at right angles to the illuminating beam – chambers may comprise flat-sided cuvettes to minimize unwanted light reflections. Water-cooled laser sources in the output power range of 50mW–5W were used for fluorescence and light-scatter measurements. Air-cooled lasers have a maximum 100mW output and are now more commonly used in commercial instruments. Lasers have the advantage of producing an intense beam of monochromatic light – the most common lasers used in flow cytometry are:

- argon lasers that produce light at wavelengths between 351 and 528nm;

- krypton lasers that produce light between 350 and 799nm;

- helium–neon lasers that produce light at 543, 594, 611 and 633nm; and

- helium–cadmium lasers that produce light at 325 and 441nm.

Light scatter and detection

Light scattered by particles as they pass through a laser or light source must be detected efficiently and fluorescent light of a given wavelength requires specific identification. The amount of light scattered is generally high in comparison with the amount of fluorescent light. Photodiodes are used therefore as forward angle light (FAL) sensors: they may be used with neutral density filters that reduce proportionally the amount of light received by the detector. To stop the laser beam and any defracted light from entering the detector a beam absorber (a diffuser or obscuration bar) is placed across the front. The scattered light is focused by a collecting lens onto the photodiode(s), which converts the photons to voltage pulses proportional to the amount of light collected (integrated pulse). These pulses may be amplified by the operator. In some systems with multiple diodes, high and low angle scattered light may be collected which may help separate populations of cells or particles.

Fluorescence analysis

Fluorescence is excited as cells traverse the laser exitation beam and is collected by optics at 90° to the incident beam. A barrier filter blocks laser excitation illumination, while dichroic mirrors and appropriate filters are used to select the required wavelengths of fluoresccence for measurement. Photons falling on the detectors are converted by photomultiplier tubes to an electrical impulse, and this signal is processed by an analogue-to-digital converter which changes the analogue impulse to a digital signal. The quantity and intensity of the fluorescence are recorded by the computer system and displayed as a frequency distribution, which may be single, dual or multi-parameter. Single-parameter histograms usually convey information regarding the intensity of fluorescence and number of cells of a given fluorescence, so that weakly fluorescent cells are distiguished from those that are strongly fluorescent. Dual-parameter histograms of forward angle scatter and 90° light scatter allow identification, based on size and granularity, of the different cell types within the preparation. Right-angle and side-scatter are alternative names used for 90° light scatter.

Aquisition

Light scatter signals may be a measure of a combination of parameters:

- size (projected surface area) of the particle;

- surface topography (i.e. rough or smooth);

- optical density (i.e. light refracted through the particle); and

- internal structure of the particle (i.e. granular or uniform).

Some of these components are present in all of the light scatter produced. The purpose of analysing the light scatter or fluorescence signal is to determine the difference between particles in terms of voltage output from detectors. There are several methods of retrieving this information:

- the maximum voltage (or peak) reached as the particle passes through the laser beam may be measured. The highest voltage reached by the pulse (pulse height) may be a measure of the maximum fluorescence given off by a particle. Particles with different amounts of associated fluorescence have different pulse heights and so peak pulses; and

- a particle with fluorescent molecules spread uniformly over the surface will produce a wide peak pulse compared with a particle with fluorescence concentrated at one point. The latter will produce a narrower and sharper peak pulse. However, the peak of the pulse may be the same for both particles and so they become indistinguishable on the basis of this parameter. The area under the two pulses will, however, be different.

The area under the pulse allows generation of a second parameter referred to as the integrated pulse. A third parameter may also be used if the width or a portion or the peak or integrated pulse is measured. This is termed time of flight (TOF).

Histograms and amplification

The production of a histogram relies on the measurement of pulses of a given value and their assignment to channels which represent different voltage levels. Each time a pulse falls in one of these channels a counter increments the channel. Most systems have 256 or 1024 channels for single-parameter histograms that may be generated on the basis of fluoresence, FAL or 90° light scatter. The pulses may be amplified either linearly or logarithmically. In some experiments the peak or integral pulses may widely vary in size. With linear amplification, small pulses will be compressed in a few channels, so making it difficult to distinguish differences between them. If the amplification is increased this helps to distinguish between the small pulses, but the larger pulses are pushed off the scale of the histogram. In such cases it is preferable to use pulses that have gone through logarithmic amplification before plotting. The plot may include all pulses. However, the small pulses will be spread over more channels and the larger pulses over fewer ones. In this way all pulses are brought within the scale of the histogram.

Once a histogram has been produced, it can be analysed. The most common analysis is to determine what percentage a subpopulation is of the total population of cells or particles. This is possible if the populations are nicely separated, but in practice it may not be the case. However, sophisticated computer programs can analyse overlapping populations. Computers can also be used to compare one histogram with another and to determine if there are any significant differences. The mean or peak channel fluorescence and the mean fluorescence intensity may also be computed and used to quantify the number of fluorescent molecules bound to the cell (see below).

Monoclonal antibodies and clusters of differentiation

A multitude of antibodies have been produced since 1975 when Kohler and Milstein introduced a method for generating clones of hybrid cells capable of producing monospecific (monoclonal) immunoglobulins in high titres. To organize these antibodies into a classification scheme there have been, to date, five international workshops whose aim has been to group the antibodies into clusters based on their cellular reactivity. These clusters have been termed clusters of differentiation or CDs of which 166 were defined at the fifth workshop in 1996.

One- and more colour immunofluorescence

- One-colour immunofluorescence is widely used to characterize functional cell types in a heterogeneous population. However, since the expression of one surface antigen is rarely unique and specific for a functional subset, this technique may be inappropriate for the discrimination between cell subsets in heterogeneous populations. This limitation may be reduced with the use of multispecific labels. In this context, two-colour immunolabelling has been used to detect double-staining of cells using the combination of two fluorochromes – fluorescein isothiocyanate (FITC) and phycoerythrin (PE) together allow good sensitivity. Both fluorochromes are excited by the 488nm line of argon lasers, with maximum emmission at 525 and 575nm for FITC and PE respectively. There is some overlap between the spectral emission of the two fluorochromes, but electronic compensation can correct for this when necessary.

- Dual-fluorescence combined with forward and 90° light scatter can provide an unambiguous identification of monocytes in normal blood. In this procedure monocytes in the lymphocyte gate are identified by their expression of CD14PE and CD45FITC. The CD45 antigen is expressed on all normal leukocytes but not on non-haemopoietic cells or mature erythrocytes. CD14 antibodies stain monocytes very brightly and have low reactivity with cells of other lineages. Thus, clear discrimination of monocytes from other cells may be made based on the surface co-expression of CD14 and CD45.

  Dual-immunofluorescence has also been used extensively to examine the expression of intracellular components in relation to cell surface molecules, for example cytoplasmic IgM, CD3, CD16 and CD22; viral antigens; and DNA content and tumour necrosis factor α. A variety of reagents has been use to permeabilize cells including ethanol, lysolecithin, and paraformaldeyde and saponin.

- Recently, antibodies coupled to fluorochromes with emission spectra >600nm have become available (e.g. Red 613, CyChrome and Quantum Red). These are based on energy transfer between two fluorochromes – phycoerythrin and cyanine-5 – and have made three-colour immunofluorescence more amenable for routine use.

Quantification of cell surface fluorescence intensity

Flow cytometry allows analysis of the level of antigen expression by individual cells. However, cellular fluorescence intensities measured by flow cytometry are generally expressed in arbitary units such that the absolute numbers of the respective cell surface determinants per antibody remain unknown. This drawback can be overcome through fluorescence quantification when using calibrated fluorescent standard beads. Fluorescence standards matched to dyes used in the test sample allow the direct conversion of the fluorescence intensity of a sample to the number of 'molecules of equivalent soluble fluorochrome' (MESF). Five calibration standards with different known levels of fluorescence are analysed using logarithmic amplification. The peak channel for each of the five standards is recorded together with the instrument settings.

The fluorescence relative channel number (RCN) for each standard is calculated from the following equations:

- for a linear amplifier:

$$RCN = \frac{\text{peak channel} \times \text{Max gain} \times 10nd;}{\text{actual gain}}$$

- for a log amplifier:

$$RCN = \text{peak channel} \times 10nd,$$

where nd is the power of the neutral density filter: nd=0 if no filter is used.

A plot of MESF (y-axis) versus RCN (x-axis) of the standards on a semilogarithmic scale provides a calibration curve that may be used to determine the MESF which corresponds to any RCN at the recorded instrument settings. Conversion of flow cytometry results to MESF allows comparison of data from different machines, and enables interlaboratory quality control.

Quantification of antibody binding to cells

The quantification of cell surface fluorescence intensity described above allows the quantification of the mean number of fluorescence equivalents associated with a given cell in a population. However, it does not provide the numbers of antibodies bound to antigens or receptors on the cell. This may be calculated by:

$$\text{Number of antibodies} = \frac{\text{average MESF,}}{\text{F:P}}$$

where F:P is the fluorochrome:protein ratio for the antibody used to identify the antigen. F:P may be determined by absorption spectroscopy at the absorption wavelength of the fluorochrome (492nm for fluorescein) and antibody (280nm for protein). However, the *F:P* determined does not translate directly to the fluorescence intensity associated with the cell because of environmental conditions. Also, quenching may occur if there are more than three fluorochrome molecules per antibody and, if the fluorochrome is ionizable, then the pH and diluent may influence fluorescence intensity. To overcome this difficulty the average fluorescence intensity per antibody (effective fluorescence F:P) is determined, instead of the number of fluorochrome molecules per antibody.

The calculation above assumes a one-to-one ratio of antibody to antigen. It should be remembered that this yields therefore only an approximation as antibody molecules are divalent and, even under saturating conditions, one molecule of antibody may bind to two molecules of antigen. In addition, the affinity of antibodies for antigens may be influenced by the concentration of the antigen, as is demonstrated by the sigmoidal curve obtained if antibody concentration is plotted against the fluorescence of bound antibody.

Cell sorting

An important function of flow cytometry is its ability to separate and collect a subpopulation of cells identified by multiparameter analysis. Classically, this sorting of cells is accomplished as the cells exit from the sample chamber in a liquid jet. Savert in 1833 showed that a stream of fluid could be broken into a series of uniform droplets when a small jet was vibrated at the appropriate frequency. In flow cytometers, the sheath stream is broken into a series of uniform droplets by vibrating the sample chamber at a high frequency with a piezoelectric crystal. Cells flowing through the flow cytometer are isolated in these tiny droplets. An electrical charge is applied to the droplet when the program detects a cell that satisfies the parameters established for sorting. The polarity of the charge – positive or negative – is determined by the sorting criteria. As the charged droplet passes an electrostatic field, it is deflected to the right or left, carrying the sorted cell with it (Fig. 3.1). Extremely pure populations of cells may be sorted at relatively rapid rates.

More recently an alternative technique has becme available for sorting cells. The FACSCalibur Sort (Becton Dickinson) employs a system where the required cell is removed from the sheath stream by a small, rotating catcher tube. Up to 300 cells s^{-1} can be sorted, but only one-way sorting is available at present. The technique is not dependent on droplet formation and takes place in an enclosed environment. Therefore, no aerosols are formed, thus reducing any risk from biohazardous samples.

CLINICAL IMPLICATIONS OF CELL ANALYSIS

Diagnostic applications of flow cytometry fall into four general categories:

- initial assessment of immune status;
- diagnosis of disease states;
- immune status following therapy and correlation with disease course; and
- molecular definition of new disease states.

Initial assessment of immune status

Flow cytometric analysis enables the enumeration of lymphocyte subsets within the total peripheral blood mononuclear cell (PBMC) population. Often blood samples are collected at one site and then shipped to another for analysis. Many options exist for the storage, preparation and staining of PBMC for flow cytometric analysis, and changes occurring during the preparatory processes (and associated delays) have been shown to result in inaccurate T cell percentages and T cell subset ratios. Preparation techniques include the conventional Ficoll-Hypaque density gradient centifugation, but this has been criticized in studies which have suggested that it:

- increased the relative proportion of B cells;

- resulted in non-viable cells being lost to the erythrocyte pellet; and

- caused selective loss of CD8+, CD57+ cells to the erythrocyte pellet.

Such difficulties have led to the development of whole-blood techniques where erythrocytes are lysed before, or after, fixation and labelling of the white blood cells occurs. Whole-blood methods also have their limitations mainly due to the effect of fixatives on antigenic epitopes and of lysing agents on cell membrane integrity. Whichever method is employed, flow cytometric analysis should be performed on fresh blood (within 2–4h of collection) without storage particularly if EDTA is used as an anticoagulant.

Ideally the process of lymphocyte gating should result in the inclusion of all lymphocytes and the exclusion of all other mononuclear cells. The presence o
f contaminating monocytes is a problem for the purposes of studying lymphocytes. Monocytes phagocytose 'foreign' particles, including fluorochrome-labelled antibodies, thus causing false-positive results. Monocytes also cause significant background reactivity with antibodies due to Fc receptor-mediated binding of antisera. However, forward and 90° light scatter parameters can be used to distinguish between lymphocytes, monocytes and neutrophils in mononuclear and whole-blood preparations. Alternatively, CD45,CD14 gating can be used as described above.

The reference distribution of peripheral blood lymphocyte subsets has been established for normal Caucasian adults, and is summarized in Table 3.1. Age and sex differences exist for some antigens, although age-related trends have been found to be similar for both sexes (at least over the 0–80-year age range). As a percentage of lymphocytes, natural killer (NK) cells and CD4+ cells increase significantly with age, while the percentage of CD8+ cells does not change significantly in adulthood. However, because the percentage of CD4+ cells increases, the CD4+/CD8+ ratio increases with age. Definite differences between sexes have been found for T cells and NK cells. Lymphocytes and NK cells of normal individuals also exhibit circadian and diurnal rhythms: for this reason, venesection in sequential studies should be undertaken on each occasion at the same time of day.

Despite changes in lymphocyte subpopulations, the sum of %T+%B+%NK approximates to 100% throughout life. The total may be >100% when dual

Table 3.1 – Reference range for major lymphocyte subsets.

Cell type	Population parameters (%)				Age variation	Sex difference
	Mean	Median	Range	SD		
CD3+ T cell	73	73	60–85	6.5	NS	2.5 F > M
CD19+ B cell	14	13	7–23	4.2	NS	NS
CD4+ T cell	44	43	29–59	7.6	1.2%/decade	3.7 M > F
CD8+ T cell	33	33	19–48	7.4	NS	NS
CD16+ CD56+ NK cell	14	13	6–29	6.0	0.9%/decade	1.6 M>F
CD4/CD8 Ratio	1.4	1.3	0.6–2.8	0.6	0.07%	0.19 F>M

SD, standard deviation; NS, not significant; M, male; F, female.

CD8+,CD4+ or CD2+,CD56+ cells are present, or when CD16+,CD56+ NK cells have been excluded from the flow-cytometric gate. Dual-positive CD4+,CD8+ lymphocytes are considered to be immature thymocytes, but increased numbers have also been found in adult T cell leukaemia, in Hashimoto's disease and thyroditis, in myesthenia gravis and thymoma, and in HTLV-1-positive T cell lymphomas. Most studies have been performed on Caucasian individuals but there is evidence for ethnic variation: for example, people of Oriental descent have relatively more NK cells, and therefore studies with such populations will require appropriate reference ranges to be determined.

Immunophenotyping results can be expressed as the absolute number of cells per microlitre of each lymphocyte subgroup, or as a percentage of the total lymphocyte population. If an aliquot of the patient's blood is analysed by a haematology counter at the same time as it is analysed by flow cytometry, the white blood cell (WBC) count and the lymphocyte differential can be determined. The absolute count for the lymphocyte subsets can therefore be calculated by:

WBC count ×% total lymphocytes ×% subset.

However, studies have shown that the medians obtained for the WBC vary greatly from site to site and for samples within the normal adult range. This variation is caused by intrinsic differences in haematology instruments produced by different manufacturers. Until the problem of comparability in absolute counts for the WBC is resolved, both percentage and local absolute values should be considered when making interpretations of lymphocyte subset population parameters. Recently, commercial kits have become available that allow the absolute number of leucocytes to be determined directly in flow cytometric samples. This is facilitated by incorporation of an internal standard of unlabelled beads at a known concentration and counting both particles and cells.

Diagnosis of disease states

The initial assessment of newly diagnosed leukaemic patients is important for identifying the type of acute leukaemia – lymphocytic or myelocytic – as this determines subsequent treatment. In most cases the classification of acute leukaemia is based on the morphology and cytochemistry of the blast cells (Table 3.2). The blasts are then categorized according to the FAB (French–American– British Co-operative group) classification (see Chapter 2 by Reid in this volume). Cytochemical techniques that use short-chain esters as substrates are widely employed for identifying cells of the monocytic and myelocytic lineage. Although monocytes usually show an intense diffuse reaction, there is increasing evidence to suggest that in clinically abnormal states (including leukaemias) this reaction may be absent. It is apparent that accurate assessment of lymphocytic, monocytic and myelocytic populations in such patients should ideally be based on a combined cytochemical–immunophenotypic approach.

Immunophenotypic analysis of leukaemias and lymphomas relies on staining patterns of the blast-cell populations with panels of antisera. Different primary panels (designed to allow distinction between myelocytic and T/B lymphocytic leukaemias) are used for acute leukaemias and chronic lymphocytic disorders. Depending on the reactivity of the blasts with the primary panel, additional panels may then be used to identify T cell subsets and monocytic, erythrocytic or megakaryocytic lineages. Table 3.3 illustrates the panels suggested by the International Committee for Standardisation in Haematology at the first Workshop on Immunophenotyping of Leukaemias and Lymphomas in 1988. More recent reports have proposed similar panals. The analysis of cytoplasmic

Table 3.2 – Differentiation of leukaemic blast cells.

	Lymphoblast	**Myeloblast**
Nucleoli	usually one	more than two
Cytoplasm	scanty high nuclear/ cytoplasmic ratio	abundant low nuclear/cytoplasmic ratio
Auer rods	absent	present
Sudan Black	negative	positive
PAS	strong block positive	negative/weak positive
Acid phosphatase	negative except in T lymphoblasts	positive
Napthol AS acetate	Negative	Positive. Myelocytic resistent to fluoride; monocytic abolished by fluoride.
Chloracetate esterase	negative	positive

Table 3.3 – Immunophenotypic panels for leukaemia diagnosis.

Cell type	Acute leukaemia Panel of antisera		Chronic lymphocytic disorders Panel of antisera	
	Primary	Secondary	Primary	Secondary
B cell	CD10 D19 cytoplasmic CD22 SIg heavy and light chains	cytoplasmic μ chain SIg μ chain	CD10 CD20 CD5 SIg heavy and light chains	CD11c CD25 CD38 FMC7
T cell	CD2 Cytoplasmic CD3 CD7	CD1 CD3 CD4 CD8	CD3	CD4 CD8 CD11b CD16 CD57
Myelocytic/ monocytic	CD13 CD33	CD14 CD15 cytoplasmic myeloperoxidase		
Erythrocytic		glycophorin A		
Megakaryocyte		CD41		
Non-specific	HLA-DR TdT	CD45 cytokeratin	HLA-DR	TdT

SIg, surface immunoglobulin; TdT, terminal deoxyribonuclear transferase.

IgM μ chains, CD3, myeloperoxidase (MPO) and nuclear TdT are usually performed on slide preparations of fixed cells. However, flow cytometric techniques have also been described for identification of IgM, MPO and TdT.

Table 3.4 – Features of acute lymphocytic leukaemia (ALL).

Feature	Null cell	Common ALL Pre-B	T ALL	B ALL
White blood cell (10⁹/l)	often <10	often >50	often >50	often <10
Cell type	L1	L1	L1 or L2	L3
Immunophenotype				
CD2	–	–	++	–
CD19	–	++	–	++
CD10	–	++	–	–
CD13	–	–	–	–
CD33	–	–	–	–
TdT	++	++	++	+/–
Incidence (%)	9	70	20	1
Karyotype	Ig and TCR gene rearrangements; always clonal			

Phenotypic analysis of the acute lymphocytic leukaemias (ALL)

An illustration of the phenotypic analysis of blood from patients with ALL is given in Table 3.4. It is clear that B cell ALLs react with CD19 and CD10, while T cell ALLs react with CD2 and TdT. Thus, different types of lymphocytic leukaemia may be distinguished. Detailed immunophenotypic and molecular analysis has shown that ALL subtypes correspond to clonal derivatives of B and T cell precursors. Equivalent normal cells proliferate in substantial numbers in foetal tissue, normal or regenerating paediatric bone marrow or thymus. Leukaemic cells, however, are not the perfect replicas of normal cells and their phenotypes may show asynchrony of gene expression. These observations accord with the view that leukaemogenesis in ALL involves an uncoupling of growth from differentiation in precursor cells, rather than a stringent maturation arrest at a precise development stage. ALL cells have diverse patterns of immunoglobulin and T cell receptor (TCR) gene rearrangements which are clonal, and ALL cells are almost always of monoclonal origin.

Phenotypic analysis of the acute myelocytic leukaemias (AML)

The immunophenotypic distinction between different myelocytic leukaemias is not so well defined (Table 3.5) with the distinction relying heavily on cytochemistry and cellular morphology. The combined use of CD13, CD33 and anti-myeloperoxidase (which detects the chain as well as the the inactive proenzyme) allows recognition of 99% of AML cases. A major contribution of CD13 and

Table 3.5 – Features of acute myelocytic leukaemias.

Feature	Immature		AML	APML	AMML	Mono	Ery	Meg
Morphology	M0	M1	M2	M3	M4	M5	M6	M7
White blood (10⁹/l)	33% less than normal				33% normal		33% above normal	
Immunophenotype								
CD2	–	–	–	–	–	–	–	–
CD19	–	–	–	–	–	–	–	–
CD10	–	–	–	–	–	–/+	–	–
CD13	+	+	+	++	++	++	–/+	–/+
CD33	+	–/+	+	++	++	++	–/+	–/+
CD14	-	–	–	–	–/+	+	–	–
CD34	++	++	+	–/+	–/+	–/+	–/+	–/+
CD68	–	–	–	–	–	–	++	–
CD41	–	–	–	–	–	–	–	+
Incidence (%)	3	70	70	7	1–2	1–2	1–2	<1

AML, acute myelocytic leukaemia; APML, acute promyelocytic leukaemia; AMML, acute myelomonocytic leukaemia; Mono. monoblastic leukaemia; Ery, erythroblastic leukaemia; Meg. megakaryocytic leukaemia.

CD33 is in the diagnosis of AML M0: in some reports – and despite evidence for the presence of myelocytic antigens – this type of leukaemia has been classified as ALL 'My' on the basis of lymphocytic morphology and negative myelocytic cyto-chemistry. It is now reasonable to classify this minimally differentiated form of AML (which represents 3% of cases) on the basis of the following features: L2 morphology; negative MPO and Sudan Black B cytochemistry; negative expression of lymphocytic antigens (although TdT and CD7 may be positive); positive expression of CD13 and/or CD33; and possible positivity for other myelocytic antigens such as CD11b, CD15 and anti-MPO. M5 may be defined by CD14 and CD68 positivity, and the M6 and M7 lineages by anti-glycophorin-A and CD41, CD42 or CD61 respectively.

Cell and chromosome sorting for the analysis of acute leukaemias

Recognition of non-random chromosome abnormalities has been an important development in the classification of acute leukaemias. These abnormalities are associated with certain forms of leukaemia defined by morphology and cytochem-istry, such as FAB types L3, M2, M3 and M5, or by immunophenotype such as early B, pre-B and B ALL. These findings led to the proposals for a classification based on morphology, immunology and cytogenetics (MIC scheme). Although all three parameters contribute to the classification of leukaemias, some types of acute leukaemias can only be defined by their karyotype (Table 3.6), and even if leukaemias may be defined without their karyotype, there is evidence that some translocations are associated with poor prognosis: pre-B ALL cases with t(1;19) have a poor prognosis. Similarly, ALLs with t(4;11) and t(9;22) are associated with very poor prognosis in adults and children. Identification of such patients is imperative as they are eligible for more radical treatment programmes, such as bone marrow transplantation. The relatively rare t(8;16) (a form of AML associated with

Table 3.6 – Chromosome translocations that define distinct types of acute leukaemia.

Translocation	Leukaemia
t(1;19)	Pre-B ALL
t(4;11)	Null ALL
t(9;22)	Ph+ ALL
t(6;9)	AML with basophilia
t(8;16)	M5 with erythrophagocytosis

In these cases the karyotype is essential when defining the leukaemia. In other known associations such as t(8;14) and L3, t(8;21) and M2, t(15;17) and M3, and t(9;11) and M5, the leukaemia is well defined by other criteria.
ALL, acute lymphocytic leukaemia; AML, acute myelocytic leukaemia.

erythrophagocytosis and coagulation features suggestive of fibrinolysis) is also associated with a low remission rate and has few long-term survivors.

Chromosomal translocations are not only important in disease classification but also have a key role in the identification of genes located at breakpoint regions and which are implicated in the pathogenesis of some leukaemias. M3 and t(15;17) are probably the best example of a well-characterized disease: the cloning and identification of the retinoic acid receptor-α (RAR-α) gene has a bearing on the differentiation and therapeutic effect obtained by ALL-*trans* retinoic acid in patients with M3.

In addition to translocations, other structural abnormalities including partial deletions and inversions can occur in leukaemic blasts. Analysis of the proteins encoded by these genes offers a new approach to understanding the consequences of the alterations which result in abnormal differentiation and proliferation of the leukaemic cells. Many of these chromosome abnormalities may be detected using the polymerase chain reaction (PCR), and flow cytometry can sort malignant cells for use in PCR and for analysis of mRNA in cells by *in situ* hybridization.

The technique of flow-sorted chromosomes has also been developed for use in fluorescent *in situ* hybridization studies. The presence of certain characteristic chromosomal translocations can be detected using breakpoint-specific probes (cosmids or yeast artifactual chromosomes – YACs), which either span or lie adjacent to such breakpoints. The same approach can be used to detect both gene deletions and amplifications when seen as homogeneously staining regions (HSRs). Whole-chromosome probe mixtures (or paints) can be used where the precise molecular nature of the event is uncertain. Chromosomal *in situ* hybridization (or painting) has been performed using Alu elements and random primer-mediated PCR products from small quantities (250–500) of flow-sorted normal and abnormal chromosomes. The Alu PCR method allows the amplification of human DNA of unknown sequence from a complex mixture of human DNA, and exploits the ubiquitous Alu repeat sequence found in such DNA: approximately 900,000 copies of this 300bp sequence are distributed in the human genome. Although there is considerable variation between copies of the Alu repeat, a consensus sequence has been established and there are regions of the repeat that are reasonably well conserved. PCR primers designed to recognize these conserved regions are used to allow inter-Alu amplification for the isolation of human DNA from complex sources. PCR products are generated from a range of normal chromosomes using the designed primers, and have been shown to be effective in *in situ* hybridization for the identification of the appropriate chromosome. This technique has been used with abnormal chromosomes and to generate region-specific paints. A consequence of this work is that chromosome paints specific for common aberrant chromosomes can be generated and made widely available for clinical use.

Analysis of biphenotypic acute leukaemia

The widespread use of monoclonal antibodies has revealed the existence of leukaemias where lymphocytic and myelocytic antigens are co-expressed on the same cells. Termed biphenotypic, they are distinct from transforming leukaemias where mixtures of lymphocytic and myelocytic cells may be present. There is considerable confusion in the literature about the definition of biphenotypic acute leukaemia: one reason is that antigens are not always critically assessed for true specificity as non-specific binding of antibodies to Fc receptors may occur. However, atypical antigen expression has been found in cases classified as AML and ALL, with perhaps a higher frequency in adults and in cases of AML.

In cases of leukaemia with biphenotypic expression, the majority of cells expresses only one, or occasionally two, inappropriate antigens such as TdT, CD2 and CD7. The lineage-specificity of these antigens is not clear. However, there is a distinct group, representing approximately 10% of all leukaemia cases and twice as frequent in cases classified as AML rather than ALL by conventional criteria, that appear to express several inappropriate antigens. In one study, 52 of 746 cases (7%) fulfilled criteria for acute biphenotypic leukaemia and consisted of four major subgroups; CD2+ AML (11 cases), CD19+ AML (8), CD13 and/or CD33+ ALL (24), and CD11b+ ALL and others (4).

A scoring system has been proposed to distinguish true biphenotypic acute leukaemias that express many antigens (including lineage-specific) from cases with minimal phenotypic deviation. The proposal is summarized in Table 3.7. A score >2 for each lineage is required to qualify the cells as biphenotypic. Most true biphenotypic cases score between 2.5 and 5. CD2 is the most frequently expressed T cell antigen in AML, and expression of this antigen has been supported by the detection of mRNA.

Table 3.7 – Scoring system for biphenotypic acute leukaemia.

	Lineage		
Points	**B cell**	**T cell**	**Myelocytic**
2	cCD22	cCD3	MPO*
1	CD10	CD2	CD13
	CD19	CD5	CD33
0.5	TdT	TdT	CD11b/c
		CD7	CD14/15

c, cytoplasmic; * demonstration of MPO by any method. To qualify as biphenotypic the score of two separate lineages should be >2.

Phenotypic analysis of lymphoproliferative disorders

Of the lymphoproliferative disorders, the B cell diseases are the most common and include chronic lymphocytic leukaemia (CLL), B cell prolymphocytic leukaemia (B PLL) and hairy cell leukaemia (HCL). The treatment modalities used for the B and T cell leukaemias are often quite different, and it is important to make the correct diagnosis. For example, B PLL does not respond to chemotherapy (chlorambucil and prednisolone) used in CLL; and HCL shows a specific response to interferon-α, deoxycoformycin and chlorodeoxyadenosine agents which are less active in CLL and B PLL. The clinical and phenotypic characteristics of these B cell leukamias are summarized in Table 3.8 together with a scoring system that has been proposed for CLL – scores range from 5 (for typical CLL) to 0 (atypical CLL).

Blood and bone marrow features resembling B cell leukaemia may develop from tissue-based non-Hodgkin's lymphoma (NHL). Involvement of blood is also seen in most cases of splenic lymphoma with circulating villous lymphocytes (SLVL), in a minority of cases of follicular lymphomas and mantle zone (intermediate or centrocytic forms), and occasionally in large cell lymphomas (Table 3.9). The importance of these disorders is two-fold:

- they present problems of differential diagnosis with other leukaemias, particularly CLL. In addition, cases of large-cell NHL often mimic morphologically acute leukaemias of the monoblastic M5 type; and

- these diseases have variable prognosis and often require a different treatment approach. For example, SLVL benefits from splenectomy, while chemotherapy is of little value.

Table 3.8 – Features of mature B cell leukaemias.

Feature	CLL	B PLL	HCL		
White blood cells (10⁹/l)	10–50 (some >50)	>50 (often <100)	<10 (rare >10)		
Monocytopenia	–	–	++		
Cell type	lymphocyte	prolymphocyte	hairy cell	Score	
				1	0
Immunophenotype*					
CD5	++	–/+	–	+	–
CD23	++	–/+	–	+	–
SmIg	–/+	++	++	–/+	++/+++
FMC7	–/+	–	++	–	++
CD22	–	++	++	–/+	++/+++

CLL, chronic lymphocytic leukaemia; PLL, prolymphocytic leukaemia; HCL, hairy cell leukaemia; * all cases positive with pan-B monoclonal antibodies, e.g. CD19, 20, 37 and HLA-DR. FMC7 has specificity for HCL.

Table 3.9 – Features of B cell non-Hodgkin's lymphoma in leukaemic phase.

Feature	Follicular lymphoma	Mantle zone	SLVL	Large cell
White blood cell (10⁹/l)	20–200	25–250	10–30	5–100
Cell type	small	medium	villous	blast-like
Immunophenotype*				
CD5	–/+	++	–	–/+
CD23	–/+	–/+	–	–
CD10	++	–/+	–/+	+
SmIg	++	++	++	++
FMC7	++	++	++	+
'M' band	–	–	++	–
Karyotype	t(14;18)	t(11;14)	t(11;14) in 20%	t(14;18) in 20%

SLVL, splenic lymphoma with circulating villous lymphocytes; * all cases positive with pan-B monoclonal antibodies, e.g. CD19, 20, 37, HLA-DR.

There are two types of leukaemias of mature T cells: T-prolymphocytic leukaemia and large granular lymphocytic leukaemia (LGL). The main features of these two disorders are given in Table 3.10 together with features of two common syndromes of mature T cells: T cell leukaemia/lymphoma and Sezary syndrome. The prognosis of most types of mature T cell leukaemias is poor with survivals of <1 year from diagnosis.

Table 3.10 – Features of mature T cell lymphomas and syndromes.

Feature	T PLL	LGL leukaemia	ATLL	Sezary syndrome
White blood cell (10⁹/l)	>100	>5	>20	>10
Neutropenia	–	++	–	–
Cell type	prolymphocytic	large granular	pleomorphic flower-like	ceribri form
Immunophenotype*				
CD7	++	+	–/+	+
CD4	++	–/+	++	++
CD8	+	++	–	–
CD25	–/+	–	++	–/+
CD56,57,11b.16	–	++	–	–
Karyotype	inv(14;18q)		variable; always clonal	

T-PLL, T cell prolymphocytic leukaemia; LGL, large granular leukaemia; ATLL, acute T lymphocytic leukaemia; * always positive with pan-T monoclonal antibodies, e.g. CD3 and CD5, and negative with CD1a and anti TdT.

Phenotypic analysis of the myeloproliferative disorders

Classification of the myeloproliferative disorders is difficult because there is a spectrum of diseases without clearly defined parameters and because one disorder is capable of transforming into another. The most prevalent disorder is chronic myelocytic (granulocytic) leukaemia (CML or CGL). The Philadelphia chromosome (Ph+) is an acquired translocation between chromosomes 22 and 9 and is highly characteristic of CML being present in 96% of cases. It is clear that AML is a disorder of stem cells common to granulocytopoiesis, erythropoiesis and probably thrombocytopoiesis, and most descendents from the diseased stem cells fail to differentiate and remain as blast cells. In CML, the progeny of the leukaemic stem cells have differentiated to some extent and may give rise to functionally useful cells. The mechanism by which useful haemopoiesis is apparently suppressed in the presence of leukaemic cells remains enigmatic. However, of those patients with CML, 80% transform to acute leukaemia – usually myelocytic leukaemia.

There are problems associated with flow cytometric immunophenotypic analysis of leukaemias. The first relates to the identification of the blast population. If the blood or bone marrow sample from the patient contains predominantly blast cells, these may be identified by atypical light-scattering properties. However, if this is not the case, dual or triple fluorescence studies may be necessary. Second, the number of blasts reactive with a given antibody is highly variable. For these reasons immunophenotyping alone (at least at present) is not sufficient to classify all leukaemias.

Diagnosis of other haematological disorders

While phenotypic analysis of lymphocytes and leukaemias is well established, similar evaluation of platelets, erythrocytes, monocytes and neutrophils may be used in the diagnosis of haematological conditions. The congenital disorders Glanzmann's thrombasthaemia (GT) and Bernard Soulier syndrome (BSS) can easily be detected based on the expression or lack of two glycoproteins (Gp): GpIIIa (CD61) and GpIb (CD42b). The platelets from patients with GT have a deficiency of the GpIIb–IIIa complex, while those from BSS patients have a deficiency of GpIb. The diagnosis of autoimmune thrombocyteopaenia (ATP) is usually made based on exclusion of other possible causes of platelet loss. The identification of platelet-associated immunoglobulin has been used in support of a diagnosis of ATP.

Paroxysmal nocturnal haemoglobinuria (PNH) is a condition with a deficiency in the molecules linked to the cell surface membrane by a glycosylphosphatydlinositol (GPI) anchor. Such molecules include decay accelerating factor (DAF, CD55) on erythrocytes; the receptor for lipopolysaccharide (CD14) on monocytes; and the Fc receptor III for human IgG (CD16) on neutrophils. The detection or lack of the molecules on blood cells by flow cytometry may be used therefore to confirm a diagnosis of PNH.

Patients with autoimmune neutropaenia (AIN), like those with ATP, are diagnosed by having a neutropaenia in isolation, neutrophil-associated immunoglobulin and with no obvious lymphocytosis. In AIN the neutropaenia may be associated with an expansion of large granular lymphocytes (LGLs). Expansion of LGLs in these patients is readily detectable by flow cytometry.

Immune status following therapy and correlation with disease course

The assessment of immune status following therapy, and correlation between immunological status and clinical course, are important in many situations. After bone marrow transplantation the patient is severely immune deficient. It is necessary, therefore, to monitor lymphocyte subpopulations to ensure that:

- a normal haemopoietic system develops;

- that onset of graft-versus-host disease is identified so that chemotherapy may be modified;

- any graft-versus-leukaemia effect in CML is monitored; and

- residual disease is detected (see below).

Recovery of lymphocyte subpopulations after bone marrow transplantation may take up to a year. The CD8+ T cell population recovers first, usually being large granular lymphocytes that exhibit NK cell activity. CD4+ T lymphocytes may not reach normal levels for at least 6 months after transplantation.

Over the past few years, peripheral blood has been used as an alternative to bone marrow for as a source of stem cells in autologous transplantation (see Chapter 1 by Bird and Marks in this issue). Levels of peripheral blood stem cells (PBSC) are increased after standard chemotherapy and after high-dose chemotherapy, such as cyclophosphamide, and the myelocytic growth factors G-CSF and GM-CSF have also been used to enhance stem cell mobilization in peripheral blood. This generation and mobilization of stem cells may be monitored by determining the % CD34+ cells in peripheral blood.

Helper and suppressor T lymphocytes have been used to correlate immune status with disease course. Although ratios significantly different from normal (0.6–2.8) have been found in many diseases, functional studies have all too often not correlated with immune imbalance perhaps because there is also a normal circadian variation (see above) and factors such as exercise which influence cell numbers. One exception is the imbalance in acquired immune deficiency syndrome (AIDS). Early in the course of this disorder, affected individuals have a reversed helper:suppressor T cell ratio due to profoundly decreased CD4+ helper cells, and this is highly predicative of clinical disease.

Analysis of cell function

It is now widely recognized that flow cytometry can be used to measure cell function, including neutrophil and monocyte phagocytosis and metabolism, cell-mediated cytotoxocity, actin polymerization, and calcium flux studies. Many of the techniques can be carried out on whole blood without the need to isolate leucocytes and, indeed, the use of whole blood may represent the preferred method for the detection and quantification of molecules associated with cell adhesion. Much interest has focused on the measurement of molecules associated with adhesion of monocytes and neutrophils, particularly during treatment with growth factors (G-CSF and GM-CSF) during stem cell transplantation. Similarly, identification of activation antigens on platelets has been investigated in a number of clinical conditions, including essential thrombasthemia, myeloproliferative disease and thrombotic conditions such as deep vein thrombosis: cellular activation correlates with disease severity.

Rare event analysis

Although one of the major advantages of flow cytometry is the ability to analyse large numbers of cells on a discrete basis, some implications of this action have not been fully appreciated until recently. Flow cytometry offers a means of quantifying minor subpopulations of cells to a degree that has been unobtainable by manual techniques. This 'rare event analysis' is limited to a frequency of 1 in 100,000, beyond which only rough estimates can be obtainable even after collecting 10^7 rare events. However, rare event analysis has been used to detect reticulocytes; malaria parasites; the survival of transfused blood cells; foetal cells in maternal blood; and, of much recent interest, the detection of CD34+ cells in recipients of PBSC transplants. Rare event analysis has also been used for the detection of minimal residual disease.

Detection of minimal residual disease

Leukaemia relapse is still the major cause of failure in the treatment of acute leukaemia. Relapse rates vary from 60 to 80% after chemotherapy, and from 20 to 50% after allogeneic or autologous bone marrow transplantation. Minimal residual disease (MRD) is defined as those relatively few leukaemic cells that have survived initial remission-induction therapy.

The total number of cells in an entire normal bone marrow compartment has been estimated to be around 10^{12}. The conventional detection level of MRD of <5% blast cells would require 10^{10} leukaemic cells to be present in the bone marrow where distribution of MRD is extremely heterogeneous. Analysis of marrow samples from different bones yields differences in leukaemic cell frequencies, so that the measured leukaemic frequency in one specific marrow sample may not reflect the concentration in other compartments. Furthermore, in man, one bone marrow aspiration contains only 0.0001% of the entire marrow compartment. Thus quantification of MRD in a given patient based on a simple bone marrow aspiration is unlikely to be successful.

Monoclonal antibodies and flow cytometry may be used to detect MRD where the presence of specific combinations of antigens on/in normal marrow cells is used to demonstrate small quantities of leukaemic cells (Table 3.11). Using such procedures it is possible to detect one leukaemic cell per 10,000 normal cells in marrow samples that were morphologically classified as coming from patients in complete remission. Furthermore, quantification of MRD correlated with the occurrence of subsequent leukaemia relapse. False-negative results in the immunological detection of MRD may be due to:

- the presence of $<10^{-4}$–10^{-5} leukaemic cells in the sample under study;

- a sampling error due to heterogeneous distribution of cells within the marrow; and

- a phenotypic switch where, in a limited number of cases, a change in phenotype has occurred between analysis at presentation and relapse.

Flow karyotyping

Conventional cytogenetic karyotypic analysis relies on the detection of chromosomal aberrations derived from metaphases (mitotic cells). Flow karyotyping has been developed where chromosomes in suspension are stained with fluorescent dyes. The dyes specifically bind to either cytosine–guanine or adenine–thymine base pairs in DNA. On excitation by dual-laser beam flow cytometers, every chromosome is individually represented in a flow karyogram. In this way numerical aberrations can be detected that are present in 40% of the acute leukaemias, and translocations that are present 10–15% of cases of ALL and in 25–30% of those with AML. In addition to conventional karyotyping, flow karyotyping offers the advan-

Table 3.11 – Detection of minimal residual disease in samples from patients morhologically in complete remission.

Cell type	Combination
T-ALL	cCD3/TdT
B-lineage-ALL	CD13/TdT CD33/TdT
Pre-B-ALL	cμ/TdT
AML	CD13/TdT CD33/TdT CD7/TdT

tage that thousands of chromosomes s^{-1} can be analysed in an objective, quantitative way, yielding a detection limit around 10^{-2} as compared with 10^{-1}–10^{-2} for conventional cytogenetic analysis. The use of fluorescence *in situ* hybridization with chromosome-specific probes has also been used on metaphase spreads, and may be performed on flow-sorted interphase cells to detect numerical aberrations and translocations. This procedure results in a detection limit of ≤10^{-3} for MRD.

CONCLUSIONS

In conclusion, flow cytometry is clearly useful in the diagnosis of a number of haematological conditions. Perhaps its most powerful contribution in the future will lie in rare event analysis. Haematology appears to be moving into an era where immunotherapy will play a role in modulating the course of diseases. Dendritic cells are receiving much interest for their use in this immunotherapy. The presence of these cells, like CD34+ stem cells, can be considered as rare events in the blood. To facilitate analysis of this rare event, manufacturers of flow cytometers are developing machines that analyse not just 20,000 but 200,000 cells s^{-1}.

SELECTED READING FOR MORE DETAILED INFORMATION

The original reference describing the production of murine monoclonal antibodies:
Kohler G, Milstein C. Continuous cultures of fused cells sectreting antibody of predefined specificity. *Nature* 1975; **256**: 495–497

Two basic references for the analysis of human peripheral blood cell numbers:
College of American Pathologists. Comprehensive Hematology Limited Coagulation Module Survey. CAP Surveys Set H1-A, 1988

Reichert T, DeBruyere M, Deneys V et al. Lymphocyte subset reference ranges in adult Caucasians. *Clinical Immunology & Immuopathology* 1991; **60**: 190–208

The original paper describing the FAB classification of acute lymphoblastic leukaemias based upon morphology:
Bennett JM, Catovsky D, Daniel MT et al. Proposals for the classification of the acute lymphoblastic leukaemias. French-American-British (FAB) Co-operative group. *British Journal of Haematology* 1976; **33**: 451–458

Three papers outlining proposals for immunophenotyping acute leukaemias:
Bennett JM, Catovsky D, Daniel MT et al. Proposal for the recognition of minimally differentiated acute myeloid leukaemia (AML-MO). *British Journal of Haematology* 1991; **78**: 325–329

Rowan RM, Bain BJ, England JM et al. Immunophenotyping in the diagnosis of acute leukaemia. *Journal of Clinical Pathology* 1994; **47**: 777–781

Scott CS, Den Ottolander GJ, Swirsky D et al. Recommended procedures for the classification of acute leukaemias. *Leukaemia Lymphoma* 1995; **18**: 1–12

Three papers on the importance of cytogenetic analysis in leukaemia diagnosis and prognosis:
Lo Coco F, Avvisati G, Diverio D et al. Rearrangements of the RAR-alpha gene in acute promyelocytic leukaemia: correlations with morphology and immunophenotype. *British Journal of Haematology* 1991; **7**: 494–499

Berger R. Cytogenetics of acute leukaemia. *Leukemia* 1992; **6** (suppl. 2): 7–11

Young BD. Advances in molecular cytogenetics: Analysis of the leukaemic cell. *British Journal of Haematology* 1992; **82**: 62–63

Three review articles highlighting the need for a leukaemia classification based on morphology, immunophenotype and cytogenetics:
Ball ED, Davis RB, Griffin JD et al. Prognostic value of lymphocyte surface markers in acute leukaemia. *Blood* 1991; **77**: 2242–2250

Catovsky D, Matutes E, Bucchrei MT et al. A classification of acute leukaemia for the 1990s. *Annals of Haematology* 1991: **62**: 16–21

Catovsky D, Matutes E. The classification of acute leukaemia. *Leukemia* 1992; **6** (suppl. 2): 1–6

Two papers describing the classification of chronic lymphoproliferative disorders:
Bennett JM, Catovsky D, Daniel MT et al. Proposals for the classification of chronic (mature) B and T cell leukaemias. *Journal of Clinical Pathology* 1989; **42**: 567–584

Catovsky D. Lymphoproliferative disorders. *British Journal of Haematology* 1992; **82**: 46–49

An important paper giving the scoring system for chronic lymphocytic leukaemia:
Matutes E, Owusa-Ankonah K, Morilla R et al. The immunological profile of B-cell disorders and proposals of a scoring system for the diagnosis of CLL. *Leukaemia* 1994; **8**: 1640–1645

An interesting paper describing the reconstitution of blood after bone marrow transplantation:
Jacobs R, Stoll M, Stratmann G et al. CD16, CD56+ natural killer cells after bone marrow transplantation. *Blood* 1992; **79**: 3239–3244

Two review articles describing stem cell transplantation and how it may be monitored:
Gale RP, Heron P, Juttner C. Blood stem cell transplants come of age. *Bone Marrow Transplantation* 1992; **9**: 151–155

Zimmerman TM, Lee JG, Bender R, Williams SF. Quantitative CD34 analysis may be used to guide peripheral-blood stem-cell harvests. *Bone Marrow Transplantation* 1995; **15**: 439–449

Two papers illustrating situations where the immune system may be altered from normal:
Fry RW, Morton AR, Crawford GP, Keast D. Cell numbers and *in vitro* responses of leukocytes and lymphocyte subpopulations following maximal exercise and interval training sessions of different intensities. *European Journal of Applied Physiology* 1992; **64**: 218–227

Katz MH, Bindman AB, Keane D, Chan AK. CD4 lymphocyte count as an indicator of delay in seeking human immunodeficiency virus-related treatment. *Archives of Internal Medicine* 1992; **152**: 1501–1504

Practical advice for users of flow cytometry in a clinical setting:
Goodall A, Macey MG. Platelet associated molecules and immunoglobulins. In Macey MG (ed.), Flow cytometry: clinical applications. Oxford: Blackwell Scientific, 1994

A good description of ways to assess minimal residual disease.
Campana D, Coustan-Smith E, Janossy G. The immunological detection of minimal residual disease. *Blood* 1990; **76**: 163–171

One of the first descriptions of the use of fluorescence in situ *hybridization for cytogenetic analysis:*
Poddighe J, Moesker O, Smeets D et al. Metaphase cytogenetics of haematological cancer: comparison of classical karyotyping and in situ hybridisation using a pannel of eleven chromosome specific DNA probes. *Cancer Research* 1991; **51**: 1959–1967

4

DETECTION AND ASSAY OF CYTOKINES: AN OVERVIEW

M. Wadhwa and R. Thorpe

SUMMARY

Accurate and sensitive methods for the measurement and detection of cytokines are an obvious prerequisite for the study of cytokine biology and biochemistry, and for the possible involvement of these molecules in pathology. In this review, the various methods available for cytokine measurement and detection (bioassays, immunoassays and other procedures) are described and compared. A critical appraisal of the potential advantages and limitations of the techniques is also included.

INTRODUCTION

Cytokines are proteins that mediate various biological effects in haemopoiesis, immunological and inflammatory responses, neuroendocrine networks, and a range of other physiological processes. More than 100 cytokines have been identified, cloned and shown to interact in complex ways to fulfil their biological functions. Perhaps not surprisingly, cytokines are also involved in both the pathogenesis and treatment of many diseases and are therefore the focus of a great deal of interest in the laboratory and clinic. Such research involves the possibility of using cytokine levels as diagnostic and prognostic markers of disease, and of the role of cytokines as therapeutic agents. The fundamental requirements for this work are accurate and sensitive assay methods for these proteins in different laboratories around the world.

PROPERTIES OF CYTOKINES

Cytokines are a diverse group of small- or medium-sized proteins or glycoproteins that show potent biological activity (Table 4.1). This activity is mediated by interaction with specific receptors on cell surfaces which trigger intracellular events leading to the biological effect. Most cytokines are produced by more than one cell type (although interleukin 3, IL-3, seems to be produced only by T cells), and act on a variety of cell types, although IL-5 is a possible exception which, in man, may act only on eosinophils. In addition, some cytokines (e.g. M-CSF and erythropoietin) show a fairly narrow range of activities, whereas others (e.g. IL-1 and IL-6) mediate a diverse range of physiological activities.

Many cytokines exist as monomeric polypeptides whereas others readily form oligomers. For example, transforming growth factor β_1 (TGFβ_1) is a homodimer,

Table 4.1 – Human cytokines – physical properties and chromosome location of the relevant gene.

Cytokine	Amino acids	MW (kDa)	Conform[1]	Glycosyl[2]	S=S no.	Chrom[3]/ gene locus
Interleukin-1α (IL-1α)	159	17.5	M	–	0	2q13–21
Interleukin-1β (IL-1β)	153	17.5	M	–	0	2q13–21
Interleukin 2 (IL-2)	133	13–17.5	M/D[4]	+(N)	1	4q26–28
Interleukin 3 (IL-3)	133	15–30	M	+(N)	1	5q23–31
Interleukin 4 (IL-4)	129	15–20	M	+(N)	3	5q31
Interleukin 5 (IL-5)	115	20–22	D	+(O & N)	0	5q23.3–32
Interleukin 6 (IL-6)	186	19–28	M	+(N)	2	7p21
Interleukin 7 (IL-7)	152	20–28	M?	+(N)	?	8q12–13
Interleukin 8 (IL-8)	72	8–10	M/D[4]	–	2	17q11.2–12
Interleukin 9 (IL-9)	126	14–25	M	+(N)	?	5q22–35
Interleukin 10 (IL-10)	160	17	M	–	2	1q31–32
Interleukin 11 (IL-11)	178	19	M	–	0	19q13.3–13.4
Interleukin 12α (IL-12α)	197	35	D	+(N)	6[5]	3p12–q13.2
Interleukin 12β (IL-12β)	306	40		+(N)	8[5]	5q31–33
Interleukin-13 (IL-13)	112	17	M	+(?)	2	5q23–31
Interleukin-14 (IL-14)	483	60	M	+(N)	?	?
Interleukin-15 (IL-15)	114	14–18	M	+(N)	2	4
Interleukin-16 (IL-16)	130	14–17	Tet	+(N)?	?	15
Interleukin-17 (IL-17)	155	15–20	D	+(N)?	?	?
Interleukin-18 (IL-18)	157	18–19	M	?	0	?
G-CSF[6]	174	18–20	M	+(O)	2	17q11.2–21
GM-CSF[7]	127	14–34	M	+(N/O)	2	5q23–31
M-CSF[8]	223	45–90	D	+(N/O)	3	1p13–21
Thrombopoietin (Tpo)	332	60–100	M	+(N)	2	3
Flt3 ligand	209	24	M	+(N)	3	19
Oncostatin M (Onco M)	196	28	M	+(N/O)	2	22
Stem cell factor (SCF)	165/248[9]	18	D	+(N/O)	2	12q14.3–qter
Erythropoietin (Epo)	166	36	M	+(N/O)	2	7q11–22
LIF[10]	180	32–62	M	+(N)	?	22q12.1–12.2
TGFβ$_1$[11]	112	12.5	D	–	5	19q13.1–13.3
TGFβ$_2$[11]	112	12.5	D	–	4	1q41
TGFβ$_3$[11]	112	12.5	D	–	4	14q23–24
Interferonα (IFNα)[12]	166	18.5	M	–	2	9p
Interferonβ (IFNβ)	166	23	M	+(N)	2	9p21
Interferonγ (IFNγ)	143	17	D	+(N)	0	12q24.1
TNFα[13]	157	17	T	–	1	6p21.1–21.3
TNFβ[13]	171	33	T	+(N)?	0	6p21.1–21.3
MCP 1,2,3[14]	76	8–17	M/D[4]	+(O)[15]	2	17q11.2–12
MIP1α[16] (LD78)	70	8	M/D[4]	–[17]	2	17q11.2–12
MIP1β[16]	69	8–12	M	?[17]	?	17q11.2–12
MIP2[16]	73?	8–10	M	?[17]	?	4?
RANTES[18]	68	8	D?	?[17]	2	17

Table 4.1 – contd.

Cytokine	Amino acids	MW (kDa)	Conform[1]	Glycosyl[2]	S=S no.	Chrom[3]
Platelet Factor 4 (PF4)	70	8	Tet	–	2	4
β-TG[19]	81	9	Tet	–	2	4q13–21
GRO/MGSA[20]	73	13–16	M	+(O)?[21]	2?	4
ENA-78	78	8	M/D	–	2	4

[[1]=Conformation; monomer (M), dimer (D), trimer (T), tetramer (Tet): [2]=Glycosylation in the N or O position: [3]=Chromosome location of gene: [4]=Conformation dependent on conditions: [5]=refers to number of intramolecular disulphide bonds; there is one intermolecular bond: [6]=Granulocyte Colony Stimulating Factor: [7]=Granulocyte Macrophage Colony Stimulating Factor: [8]=Macrophage Colony Stimulating Factor: [9]= Number of amino acids varies for the membrane-bound and soluble forms: [10]=Leukemia Inhibitory Factor: [11]=Transforming Growth Factor: [12]=Many similar forms identified each the product of separate genes: [13]=Tumour Necrosis Factor: [14]=Monocyte Chemoattractant Proteins 1,2,3: [15]=O-linked glycosylation present in MCP-1 only; no glycosylation in MCP-2; unknown for MCP-3: [16]=Macrophage Inflammatory Protein: [17]=No sites for N-linked glycosylation: [18]=Regulated on Activation, Normal T Expressed and Secreted: [19]=β-Thromboglobulin: [20]=Melanoma Growth Stimulatory Activity: [21]=No N-linked glycosylation but potential sites for O-linked glycosylation. Information compiled by Wadhwa & Thorpe, and Pallister & Marriott (Chapter 5).]

whereas IL-12 is a heterodimer. Tumour necrosis factor α (TNFα) is an exception as it occurs primarily as a trimer (Table 1). Some cytokines are produced as larger precursor molecules processed by enzyme-mediated proteolysis to smaller molecular weight forms: in some cases, the precursor is essentially biologically inactive (e.g. IL-1β), whereas other precursors have significant biological activity (such as the 31 Kd IL-1α precursor). M-CSF is rather unusual as it can be produced as 'long' or 'short' biologically active forms depending on which spliced variant of mRNA is used for translation. Some cytokines have typical leader amino acid sequences that are necessary for secretion from cells and which are cleaved during this process: others, such as IL-1 and TNFα, do not appear to possess such leader structures and their mechanism of secretion from cells remains obscure. Although many cytokines are glycosylated, the carbohydrate chains are not necessary for biological activity at least in most *in vitro* systems. However, glycosylation can affect the pharmacokinetics of cytokines and for some this can be very important for correct *in vivo* function (e.g. erythropoietin: see Chapter 7 by Dunn and Marriott in this issue). In some cases, cytokines from one species are biologically active on cells from most other (at least mammalian) species (e.g. IL-1 and G-CSF): in other cases (e.g. IL-4, IL-3 and GM-CSF) fairly strict species specificity is exhibited although most human cytokines act effectively on other primate cells. A few cytokines such as IL-2 and IL-6 show an interesting 'one way' restriction of species specificity – the human cytokines efficiently stimulate rodent cells, but the murine molecules are completely inactive in human systems. Some cytokines, such as TNFα and interferon γ (IFNγ), show a graded decline in biological activity as the evolutionary distance of cytokine and responding cell(s) increases.

PRODUCTION OF CYTOKINES

Cytokines are secreted by many cell types, usually following some form of stimulus. Most investigations on cytokines have concentrated on mammalian systems, but evidence suggests that molecules with cytokine-like activity exist in lower animals. In most cases fairly low levels of cytokines are produced, and usually more than one cytokine is produced following stimulation – observations which handicapped the detailed and specific study of cytokines for a considerable period. However, the use of molecular biology and rDNA procedures has allowed the identification, cloning and expression of cytokine genes which, in turn, has permitted in-depth study of cytokine biology and biochemistry, and the production of relatively large quantities of 'clinical grade' material suitable for therapeutic use in man. Several cytokines have been successfully developed as therapeutic agents, e.g. IL-2, G-CSF, erythropoietin (Epo), GM-CSF, IFNα and IFNβ.

ASSAYS FOR CYTOKINES

Various types of assays are now available for the estimation of cytokines present in a wide range of biological fluids. Often the biological activities elicited by a particular cytokine become the basis for its biological detection and assay, e.g. formation of granulocyte colonies by G-CSF. Such bioassays have been complemented by the development of immunoassays or alternative immunochemical or biochemical techniques for the measurement and identification of cytokines.

Bioassays for cytokines

Numerous bioassays using either whole animals *in vivo* or isolated cells *in vitro* have been developed for the quantitation of cytokines. Whole animal assays provide invaluable information about the biological activity of cytokines as well as a useful assessment of their biological potency. Common examples of this type of assay are the pyrogen assay for IL-1 and the post-hypoxic polycythaemic mouse assay for Epo. However, such assays are now seldom used and have been largely superseded by *in vitro* bioassays using either primary cell cultures (Tables 4.2 and 4.3) or continuous cell lines (Table 4.4).

Cells of the haemopoietic or immune systems isolated from bone marrow, blood, or other tissues or organs/glands (e.g. liver, spleen, thymus, etc.) from human or other animal sources are often used in the early stages of research with newly identified cytokines. These assays are very useful for showing biological effects of particular cytokine. For example, the bone marrow colony assay for assessment of colony-stimulating activity is useful when examining the effects of individual cytokines or a combination of cytokines on haemopoiesis *in vitro*. In certain instances, purified cell populations (e.g. B or T lymphocytes, monocytes, neu-

Table 4.2 – Whole animal and primary cell culture-based assays for cytokines.

Cytokine	Target system	Biological assay
IL-1	thymocytes fibroblasts skeletal explants synovial cells hepatocytes *in vivo* – mouse/rat *in vivo* – mouse/rabbit	mitogenesis cytokine induction (e.g. IL-6) bone resorption release of collagenase or PGE_2 induction of acute phase proteins induction of acute phase proteins pyrogen assay
IL-2	mitogen-activated T cells	proliferation
IL-3	bone marrow progenitor cells	formation of haematopoietic mixed colonies
IL-4	B cells stimulated with either SAC, anti-Ig or anti-CD40 monoclonal antibodies or phorbol esters Tonsillar cells	proliferation assay Enhancement of activation antigens (e.g. CD23) or surface IgM expression
IL-5	bone marrow	formation of eosinophil colonies or estimation of eosinophil peroxidase
IL-6	B cells stimulated with anti-CD40 monoclonal antibodies hepatocytes	enhancement of IgG secretion induction of acute phase proteins
IL-7	precursor B cells mitogen-stimulated T cells	proliferation proliferation
IL-9	long-term culture of activated peripheral blood lymphocytes bone marrow mast cells/cell lines	proliferation formation of erythroid colonies in the presence of Epo proliferation
IL-10	activated peripheral blood mononuclear cells, mitogen-activated Th1 clones mast cells macrophages	inhibition of IFNγ production enhancement of IL-3/IL-4-induced proliferation inhibition of cytokine production following activation by lipopolysaccharide (LPS)
IL-11	bone marrow B cells	stimulation of megakaryocyte colony formation in synergy with IL-3 proliferation

Table 4.2 – contd.

Cytokine	Target system	Biological assay
IL-12	PHA-activated lymphoblasts NK cells NK cells	proliferation stimulation of IFNγ production augmentation of NK cell activity
IL-13	monocytes B cells co-stimulated with anti-Ig and anti-CD40 antibodies	upregulation of MHC class II expression inhibited production of inflammatory cytokines in response to LPS/IFNγ proliferation
IL-14	B cells activated with SAC	proliferation
IL-15	Activated T lymphocytes B cells NK cells	proliferation proliferation activation
IL-16	T cells	chemotaxis assay
IL-17	T cells fibroblasts	proliferation secretion of cytokines (e.g. IL-6, G-CSF)
IL-18	peripheral blood mononuclear cells	induction of IFNγ production augmentation of NK cell activity
G-CSF	bone marrow bone marrow neutrophils	formation of granulocyte colonies proliferation enhancement of superoxide production
GM-CSF	bone marrow monocytes/granulocytes neutrophils	formation of granulocyte macrophage colonies increased expression of adhesion molecules respiratory burst activity
M-CSF	bone marrow monocytes	macrophage colony formation production of cytokines (e.g. IFN, TNF)
Tpo	bone marrow	formation of megakaryocyte colonies
Flt3 ligand	bone marrow/foetal liver	synergy with CSFs in multilineage colony formation

Table 4.2 – contd.

Cytokine	Target system	Biological assay
SCF	bone marrow/cord blood	synergy with CSFs and other cytokines in multilineage colony formation
	mast cells	proliferation
Epo	*in vivo* post-hypoxic polycythaemic mouse	stimulation of erythropoiesis
	bone marrow	formation of erythroid colonies
LIF	bone marrow	synergy with IL-3 in megakaryocyte colony formation
TNFα/β	endothelial cells	induction of HLA class I expression, increased expression of adhesion molecules
	hepatocytes	upregulation of acute phase proteins
	fibroblasts	proliferation
	synovial cells	production of collagenase and PGE_2

trophils, etc.), are used for proliferation assays, or assays of respiratory burst, chemotaxis, natural killer (NK) cell stimulatory activity, etc., and can provide a quantitative estimate of cytokine levels. However, a drawback of such bioassays is that results can be difficult to reproduce because of variation between donors, and the complexity of preparing purified cell preparations.

As an alternative to primary cell cultures, continuous cell lines and/or transfected lines derived either from laboratory-induced leukaemias or from leukaemic patients are often used in bioassays. Such cell-line based assays are economical, easy to use and analyse, and generally produce reliable, reproducible and accurate estimates of biologically active cytokine. However, these assays also have inherent limitations.

A major problem is that cell-line based assays are seldom specific for a single cytokine. For example, the TF-1 erythroleukaemia cell line proliferates in response to a range of cytokines, and is also susceptible to cytokines such as TGFβ, IFNα and IFNβ which inhibit the proliferative response to stimulatory cytokines. In certain instances, bioassays may underestimate the cytokine activity in biological samples due to the presence of inhibitors, e.g. IL-1 receptor antagonist, soluble cytokine receptors. Alternatively, these bioassays may overestimate cytokine content due to synergistic interactions between individual cytokines. Interpretation of the results obtained for cytokine content in biological fluids is therefore difficult as the measured proliferation could be due to antagonistic/synergistic interactions between one or more cytokines present in variable proportions (Table 4.4). One approach to identify the specific cytokine eliciting the response is to use antibodies specifically to neutralize the effects of single cytokines.

Table 4.3 – Primary cell culture-based assays for cytokines.

Cytokine	Target cells in chemotaxis assay	Other assays
IL-8	neutrophils, basophils, T cells	degranulation of neutrophils respiratory burst activity and lysosomal enzyme release from neutrophils induction of Ca^{2+} fluxes in monocytes release of histamine from basophils
MCP 1,2,3	monocytes, basophils	induction of histamine release from basophils augmentation of superoxide poduction and lysosomal enzyme release from monocytes
MIP1α	monocytes, B cells, cytotoxic, T cells, CD4+ T cells, basophils, eosinophils	induction of histamine release from basophils and mast cells stem cell inhibition induction of Ca^{2+} fluxes in monocytes
MIP1β	monocytes, CD4+ T cells (preferentially the 'naive' T cells)	lysosomal enzyme release and degranulation of neutrophils
RANTES	monocytes, eosinophils, basophils, memory T cells	induction of histamine release from basophils
PF4	monocytes, neutrophils, fibroblasts	inhibition of angiogenesis
β-TG	neutrophils, fibroblasts	
GRO/MGSA	neutrophils	induction of Ca^{2+} fluxes in monocytes induction of respiratory burst activity and lysosomal enzyme release from neutrophils
ENA-78	neutrophils	induction of Ca^{2+} fluxes in neutrophils
I-309	monocytes	induction of Ca^{2+} fluxes in monocytes
IP-10	monocytes, T cells	
NAP-2	neutrophils	induction of Ca^{2+} fluxes in neutrophils elastase release from neutrophils

Table 4.4 – Cell line-based assays for cytokines.

Cytokine	Cell line	Origin	Endpoint	Range (/ml)	Other cytokines
IL-1	D10S	murine T-helper cell	proliferation	0.01–10IU	IL-2
	A375	human melanoma	inhibition of proliferation	0.01–10IU	TNFα, TNFβ, TGFβ_1, TGFβ_2, IL-6, LIF
	NOB-1	murine thymoma	production of IL-2		TNF
IL-2	CTLL-2	murine cytotoxic T cell	proliferation	0.01–10IU	IL-15, TGFβ_1, TGFβ_2
	KIT-225	human chronic T lymphocytic leukaemia	proliferation	0.1–20IU	IL-12, IL-7, IL-15
IL-3	MO7e	human megakaryoblastic leukaemia	proliferation	0.05–20IU	GM-CSF, SCF, IL-9, IL-15, Tpo, TNFα, TNFβ, IFNα, IFNβ, TGFβ_1, TGFβ_2
	TF-1	human erythroleukaemia	proliferation	0.02–10IU	IL-4, IL-5, IL-6, IL-13, IL-15, GM-CSF, NGF, SCF, LIF, Onco M, CNTF, Epo, TNFα, TNFβ, IFNα, IFNβ, TGFβ_1, TGFβ_2
IL-4	CT.h4S	murine cytotoxic T cell transfected with hIL-4	proliferation	0.1–25IU	IL-2, TNFα, TNFβ, IFNα, IFNβ, TGFβ_1, TGFβ_2
	CCL-185	human lung tumour	inhibition of proliferation	0.05–10IU	IL-13, IL-1, TNFα, TNFβ
	RAMOS	human B cell lymphoma	augmentation of CD23 expression	1–20IU	TNFα, TNFβ
IL-5	TF-1	as above	proliferation	0.1–50IU	as above
IL-6	B9	murine hybridoma	proliferation	0.05–5IU	IL-13, IL-11
	CESS	human B cell	production of IgG	20–5000IU	
	7TD1	murine hybridoma	proliferation	0.1–15IU	
IL-7	2bx	murine pre-B cell	proliferation	10–5000U	IL-2, IL-12, IL-15
	KIT-225	as above	proliferation	5–1000U	

Table 4.4 – contd.

Cytokine	Cell line	Origin	Endpoint	Range (/ml)	Other cytokines
IL-9	MO7e	as above	proliferation	0.5–100U	as above
IL-10	MC-9	murine mast cell line	proliferation	1–100U	IL-5
	Bac8.1c1	murine pro-E cells transfected with hIL-10 receptor	proliferation	0.5–500U	
IL-11	B9–11	murine hybridoma	proliferation	0.2–50U	IL-6, IL-13
	T10	murine plasmacytoma	proliferation	0.5–50U	IL-6
IL-12	KIT-225	as above	proliferation	0.01–20U	IL-2, IL-7, IL-15
IL-13	B9.1.3	murine hybridoma	proliferation	0.3–20U	IL-6, IL-11
	TF-1	as above	proliferation	0.5–100U	as above
IL-15	CTLL-2	as above	proliferation	0.2–10U	as above
	KIT-225	as above	proliferation	1–1000U	IL-2, IL-7, IL-12
G-CSF	GNFS-60	murine myeloid leukaemia	proliferation	0.5–100IU	IL-6, $TGF\beta_1$, $TGF\beta_2$, M-CSF, Onco M, LIF, IL-13
	WEHI3BD+	murine myelomonocytic leukaemia	differentiation	10–100IU	GM-CSF
GM-CSF	MO7e	as above	proliferation	0.1–10IU	as above
	TF-1	as above	proliferation	0.01–5IU	as above
M-CSF	MNFS-60	murine myeloid leukaemia	proliferation	1.5–150IU	IL-6, $TGF\beta_1$, $TGF\beta_2$, G-CSF, Onco M, LIF, IL-13
	BAC1.2F5	SV40-transformed murine macrophage ine	proliferation	10–100IU	GM-CSF

Table 4.4 – *contd.*

Cytokine	Cell line	Origin	Endpoint	Range (/ml)	Other cytokines
Tpo	MO7e	as above	proliferation	20pg-20ng	as above
	32D/Mpl+	murine myeloid leukaemia transfected with the formpl receptor	proliferation	20pg-2ng	as above
Onco M	A375	human melanoma	inhibition of proliferation	0.5-100U	IL-1, IL-6, LIF, TNFα, TNFβ, TGFβ$_1$, TGFβ$_2$
	TF-1	as above	proliferation	0.5-500U	as above
SCF	MO7e	as above	proliferation	1-100U	as above
	TF-1	as above	proliferation	1-100U	as above
Epo	UT-7/EPO	megakaryoblastic leukaemia	proliferation	200pg-10ng	TGFβ$_1$, TGFβ$_2$
	TF-1	as above	proliferation		as above
LIF	DA-1a	murine myeloid leukaemia	proliferation	0.01-100U	G-CSF
	TF-1	as above	proliferation	0.05-50U	as above
TGFβ	MuLv1	mink lung fibroblasts	proliferation	10pg-1ng	TNFα, TNFβ
	TFl	as above	inhibition of proliferation	500fg-1ng	as above
IFNα	2D9+EMCV	human glioblastoma + encephalomycarditis virus	anti-viral	0.1pg-2pg	IFNβ
	TF-1	as above	inhibition of proliferation	0.5pg-10ng	as above
	Daudi	human B lymphoblastoid	inhibition of proloferation	1-100pg	

Table 4.4 – *contd.*

Cytokine	Cell line	Origin	Endpoint	Range (/ml)	Other cytokines
IFNβ	2D9+EMCV	as above	anti-viral	0.3–6pg	IFNα
	TF-1	as above	inhibition of proliferation	0.5pg–10ng	as above
	Daudi	as above	inhibition of proliferation	10pg–1ng	
IFNγ	2D9+EMCV	as above	anti-viral	20–200pg	as above
	COLO205	human colorectal carcinoma	MHC class II expression	20–2000pg	
TNFα	KYM-1D4	human rhabdomyosarcoma	cytotoxicity	0.2–4IU	none
	L-M	murine fibroblast	cytotoxicity	0.2–4IU	
	WEHI164	human fibrosarcoma	cytotoxicity	0.04–2IU	
TNFβ	KYM-1D4	as above	cytotoxicity	4–75IU	
	WEHI164	as above	cytotoxicity	0.075–40IU	
	L-M	murine fibrob asts	cytotoxicity	0.10–30IU	
MCP 1,2,3	THP-1	human acute monocytic leukaemia	chemotaxis	0.02–100U	RANTES, MIP-1α
MIP-1α	THP-1	as above	chemotaxis	0.2–10U	RANTES, MCP 1,2,3
RANTES	THP-1	as above	chemotaxis	0.02–10U	MIP-1, MCP 1,2,3
GRO/MGSA	Hs294T	human melanoma	proliferation	100pg–100ng	IL-8
	U937	human monocytic	Ca²⁺ mobilization	10–1000ng	IL-8

Another limitation of bioassays is their dependence on retained characteristics of cell lines: some cell lines become spontaneously independent of a requirement for the particular cytokine being assayed, thus requiring frequent subcloning and monitoring for sensitivity and specificity. In some cases, it is possible to increase specificity by using cell lines from a different species from the source of the cytokine. For example, the mouse CTLL-2 cell line proliferates in response to both murine and human IL-2, and murine IL-4, but is unresponsive to human IL-4, and can therefore be used specifically to measure human IL-2 in biological samples. The approach of transfecting cytokine receptors into continuous cell lines has produced several specific lines such as CT.h4S cells for the assay of IL-4 and 32D/Mpl+ for thrombopoietin but it is possible that these cell lines may still retain responsiveness to other cytokines.

Proliferation and anti-proliferation bioassays

In such assays, cytokine levels are estimated simply by their ability to stimulate or inhibit cellular proliferation. Effects on proliferation rate can be assessed by several methods of which tritiated thymidine (^{3}H-TdR) incorporation into DNA is probably most commonly used. Non-radioactive procedures using an index of cell metabolism as a surrogate for cell proliferation are becoming increasingly popular. Thus, tetrazolium salts such as MTT, XTT, MTS and WST-1 are useful for measuring proliferation of lymphokine-dependent cell lines. Detection of metabolic products (e.g. ATP, cAMP) by bioluminescence can also be used. As with ^{3}H-TdR-based systems, automated systems have been devised to deal with non-radioactive procedures.

Induction of cell surface molecules

Alterations in expression of specific cell surface molecules can be used to bioassay some cytokines. Such assays have been based on upregulation of MHC class I molecules by IFNγ on various cell types; CD23 on B cells or cell lines by IL-4; or expression of cellular adhesion molecules, e.g. ICAM-1 on glioblastoma or astrocytoma cell lines with cytokines such as IL-1α/β, TNFα/β and IFNγ. In these assays, the biological response can be quantified immunochemically by microscopy or by flow cytometry, or alternatively with ELISAs or IRMAs (see below).

Induction of secretion of 'secondary' molecules

The ability of some cytokines to enhance or inhibit secretion of some substances from appropriate cell types can form the basis of a bioassay (Tables 4.2–4.4). For example, IL-6 can be measured by its ability to enhance IgG secretion by some B cell or plasmacytoma cell lines, or by synthesis and secretion of acute-phase proteins such as 1-antichymotrypsin from hepatoma cell-lines or hepatocytes. IL-1 can be determined by its ability to induce secretion of IL-2 from T cells. Some cytokines inhibit secretion of other cytokines sufficiently for this phenomenon to be used for their assay. Thus, IL-10 can be determined by its ability to inhibit IFNγ. Some cytokines, e.g. GM-CSF and IL-8, induce neutrophil degranulation measured by release of granule constituents such as β-glucuronidase, elastase or myeloperoxidase, and this can form the basis of their assay.

Anti-viral assays

The potent anti-viral activity of some cytokines, e.g. the IFNs, constitutes the basic principle of these assays. Susceptible cells are incubated with IFN prior to the addition of a cytopathic virus, and the number of viable cells are subsequently estimated either by ^{3}H-TdR incorporation, tetrazolium salt reduction or vital stains such as napthol blue-black or neutral red. Generally, various combinations of target cells such as primary human fibroblasts or cell-lines (e.g. 2D9, Hep 2C, WISH, A549) and challenge viruses (Encephalomycarditis virus, Vesicular stomatitis virus, Semliki Forest virus) are available for anti-viral assays with some combinations providing accurate, sensitive and reliable results.

Bone marrow colony-formation assays

Assessing bone marrow colony-formation remains the definitive assay for the CSFs. In this technique bone marrow cells are cultured in soft agar with dilutions of CSFs. After 7–14 days, the numbers or colonies obtained are counted with the colony number being directly related to the concentration of CSF. Staining of dried and fixed culture gels allows identification of the cell types in colonies with the colony type being highly dependent on the stimulating factor: IL-3 and GM-CSF stimulate the production of mixed colonies of different cell lineages, while cytokines such as G-CSF and M-CSF tend to be more restrictive and stimulate colonies of only one cell type. These assays are time-consuming, tedious, require considerable skill to perform consistently and can be easily influenced by contaminating factors which may enhance or inhibit colony formation. In addition, the assay end-point (size and type of colony) is very subjective and automated methods are not yet reliable.

Cytotoxic assays

Some cytokines, notably TNFα and TNFβ are assayed by their potent cytotoxic effect on susceptible cell lines (Table 4.4). In these assays, cells (usually as an adherent monolayer) are cultured with dilutions of cytokine, and the cytotoxic activity assessed by uptake of a dye, e.g. naphthol blue-black, and quantified using an optical reader. The amount of dye associated with the cells is proportional to the number of viable cells, which is inversely proportional to cytotoxic activity. For partially adherent and non-adherent cells, alternative methods that employ ^{3}H-TdR or tetrazolium salts can be used.

Inhibition of cytokine activity

Some cytokines inhibit the activity of other cytokines to such an extent and with such specificity that this inhibition constitutes the basis of an assay. For example, TGFβ-mediated inhibition of the proliferative effects of IL-5, and IFN-mediated inhibition of the proliferative effects of GM-CSF.

Chemotaxis assays

For chemokines, the only suitable biological assays are often those based on chemotaxis where cytokine levels are quantified by their ability to attract cells through membranes. Several commercially available chambers can be used for chemotaxis assays, and those that incorporate a standard 96-well microtitre plate are most appropriate. Cell number can be measured by any of the methods described previously.

Assessment of respiratory burst induction

Some cytokines (e.g. IL-8 and TNF) can be measured by their ability to induce a respiratory burst in neutrophils. GM-CSF primes neutrophils for a potent respiratory burst, which can be triggered by other molecules such as fmet-leu-phe. The effect can be measured in neutrophils by spectrophotometric estimation (at 550nm) of the reduction of cytochrome C by release of superoxide anions.

Measurement of ionic flux

Measurement of a cytokine-mediated calcium flux using appropriate fluorescent calcium indicator dyes (quin 2, fura 2, indo 3) can be used as an assay for some cytokines, particularly members of the chemokine family.

Reporter gene-based assays

In these assays, appropriate cells are transfected with constructs consisting of the promoter of a gene known to be induced by the cytokine fused to a reporter gene system. On the basis of this approach, an assay has been described for TGFβ using a truncated plasminogen activator inhibitor-I promoter fused to the gene for firefly luciferase. Addition of TGFβ to the cells induces a dose-dependent increase in the secretion of luciferase, which can be quantified using either tritium-labelled substrates or chromogenic procedures.

Kinase receptor activation assay (KIRA)

KIRA is a recent development in the assay of cytokines. In this procedure, the interaction of the cytokine with its receptor triggers phosphorylation of a specific protein, the levels of which can be detected using an appropriate and sensitive immunoassay.

Immunoassays for cytokines

Immunoassays provide a convenient method for cytokine measurement and are usually easier and quicker to perform than bioassays. They can be used to distinguish cytokines that have similar biological activities, e.g. IL-1α and IL-1β, TNFα, and TNFβ.

Most cytokine immunoassays follow established techniques including radioimmunoassays (RIAs), immunoradiometric assays (IRMAs) and enzyme-linked immunosorbent assays (ELISAs). Conventional competitive binding RIAs are not usually sufficiently sensitive to measure physiological or even pathological levels of cytokines. Furthermore, when used for assaying cytokines in complex biological fluids they are often subject to so-called 'matrix effects' which necessitate some kind of sample extraction prior to assay. Use of different immunoassay formats involving different antibodies and standards can result in considerable variation in immunoassay estimates of a single cytokine preparation.

The most useful immunoassays are those based on a 'two-site' principle – one antibody captures the cytokine antigen(s), and another, suitably labelled, detects bound antigen. This format can be particularly specific if at least one of the antibody pair is a carefully characterized monoclonal antibody. Such assays can be used to measure cytokines in complex biological fluids without pretreatment of samples, and can be either IRMAs or ELISAs using radiolabelled or enzyme-labelled detector antibodies respectively. A problem that sometimes occurs with two-site assays is that immobilization of 'capture' antibody causes steric changes which severely compromises subsequent binding events essential for the assay. One possible solution to this difficulty is to modify the procedure to allow antibody recognition to occur in liquid phase followed by capture of antibody–antigen (cytokine) complexes with a solid phase anti-immunoglobulin reagent. Some ELISA methods have been coupled to enzyme amplification cascades which claim to increase sensitivity.

A significant problem with immunoassays for cytokines (and other biological materials) is that they can detect biologically inactive or partially active molecules. This problem can be particularly important when analysing complex biological samples, and may result in a significant and variable lack of correlation between the biological activity of a particular cytokine (detected by bioassay) and the quantity of cytokine estimated using immunoassays. The loss of biological activity can be due to denaturation by proteases, or other factors such as complexing with inhibitors like soluble cytokine receptors. Incorrect folding or refolding of rDNA-derived molecules can also influence biological activity.

Another problem with immunoassays is that, because of variable recognition of cytokine subspecies by the antibodies, they may have a differential sensitivity for different subforms of the cytokine. Factors such as variable glycosylation, amidation, primary structure (both those intentionally introduced in rDNA-derived materials and naturally occurring) and differences in secondary, tertiary or even quaternary structure can influence the interaction of cytokine molecules with antibodies and therefore the results obtained using immunoassays. These effects can be 'all or none' (a particular antibody either reacts well or will not bind at all to a particular subspecies), or may be graded in effect between different cytokine forms. The result of this phenomenon is that a particular immunoassay can fail to detect a particular form of a cytokine, whereas other forms are detected in amounts that variably reflect the total or partial biological activity of cytokine preparations. This results in an overall assessment of cytokine content that can be unrelated to biological activity, and which will vary according to the precise subspecies composition of different preparations

Immunoassays can also be influenced by 'matrix effects' when used for estimating the cytokine content of some biological fluids, e.g. serum, plasma, etc. As with all immunoassays, the specificity, sensitivity and other characteristics relating to the quality of the procedure are mainly determined by the particular antibodies used. Use of different immunoassay formats involving different antibodies and standards can result in a very considerable variation in immunoassay estimates of a single cytokine preparation.

Receptor binding assays

Receptor binding assays can be used to assess levels of cytokine molecules able to interact with cytokine receptors. Cytokine receptor molecules (often produced using rDNA technology) can be used in place of the capture antibody; the assays have the advantage that such receptors usually have very high affinities for appropriate cytokines, and they are, with some exceptions, very specific and do not detect aberrant or degraded cytokine molecules which have lost the ability to react with receptors and induce biological effects. Such assays can in some cases be regarded as intermediate between bioassays and immunochemical assays. However, the results obtained using receptor binding assays (especially those using isolated or rDNA-produced receptor molecules) may not correlate with data generated using bioassays. This is because some cytokine molecules appear to bind to receptors but cannot 'trigger' the receptor to initiate the signal transduction mechanism essential for production of the biological effect. Receptor-based assays using other formats, e.g. competitive displacement assays using receptor bearing cells, have also been devised for cytokine detection.

DETECTION OF CYTOKINES IN CELLS AND TISSUES

Although bioassays or immunoassays are useful for examining cytokine production at the cell population level, they do not provide information concerning the frequency and cell surface phenotype of individual cytokine-producing cells. In recent years, however, specific procedures have been developed to estimate cytokine production at the level of an individual cell. Such procedures include the enzyme-linked immunospot 'ELISPOT' procedure, and reverse haemolytic plaque assays (RHPA).

In ELISPOT, single cells are overlaid on immobilized cytokine-specific antibody (usually in tissue culture plates). After a suitable incubation period, the secreted cytokine molecules are 'captured' by the antibody and detected by routine immunocytochemical methods using enzyme-labelled, cytokinc-specific antibody followed by an appropriate substrate. This technique has been used to detect and enumerate human lymphocytes secreting IFNγ, and human cells from kidney allografts secreting IFNγ, IL-6 and IL-10. For RHPA, a similar strategy is adopted as for ELISPOT except protein A-treated red blood cells coated with appropriate cytokine-specific antibodies are used for detection of secreted cytokine molecules from individual cells. In the ELISPOT technique, cytokine-secreting cells are identified by spots of chromogenic substrate, whereas plaques of haemolysis are produced by cells in the RHPA procedure. The diameter of the plaques in RHPA is usually approximately proportional to the amount of cytokine produced by secreting cells, and this approach has been used to quantify the release of various cytokines by human blood and tumour-infiltrating leukocytes. An alternative method for identification of cytokine-secreting cells is cell-blotting, which is based on passive adsorption of secreted cytokines to a protein-binding membrane followed by immunocytochemical detection.

Information regarding the tissue or cellular localization of cytokines can also be obtained by direct immunofluorescent techniques, or with flow cytometry/fluorescence microscopy coupled to image analysers. Double labelling methods combining cytokine-specific antibodies with antibodies that detect surface markers or non-cytokine cytoplasmic proteins provide information on the cell types that synthesize cytokines and the antigens co-produced with them. The development of various immunostaining methods now facilitates the identification of producer cells, allows visualization of production of more than one cytokine within an individual cell, aids investigation of receptor expression and, in some instances, is even capable of distinguishing the subcellular organelles involved in cytokine synthesis.

The success of the ELISPOT and RHPA methods depends on the selection of suitable fixatives and cell-permeabilizing agents (i.e. paraformaldehyde and saponin) that both maintain cell morphology and cytokine epitope configurations, and provide access to antigenic forms of immobilized intracellular cytokines with minimal cell aggregation or loss. However, a serious drawback to these procedures is that high 'background', artefactual staining is often seen with many antibodies and it is essential that antibody specificity is demonstrated by preincubating the putative cytokine-specific antibody with an excess of corresponding recombinant cytokine. Another problem is that the procedures may not be sufficiently sensitive to detect cytokines unless they are present in abnormally high amounts.

It is now possible to detect simultaneously not only the translated cytokine product and/or the phenotype of the producer cell, but also to use reverse transcriptase-polymerase chain reaction (RT-PCR) to demonstrate cellular cytokine mRNA expression. Detection of cytokine transcripts in individuals cells by RT-PCR is a very useful technique for assessing the levels of cytokine mRNA as it provides an indication of the level of localized cytokine synthesis. However, production of cytokine mRNA and protein may not necessarily be correlated. In addition, a particular cytokine associated with a given cell may not have been synthesized by that particular cell, but may represent an internalized product of another cell type. Besides RT-PCR, various *in situ* hybridization procedures involving the use of appropriately radio- or enzyme-labelled oligonucleotide probes can be used for detection of cytokine mRNA, but such procedures are also associated with their own set of difficulties.

SAMPLE PREPARATION

If artefacts are to be avoided, the preparation and collection of samples intended for cytokine assays is critically important. Cytokine levels are often measured in culture supernatant or biological fluids such as serum, plasma or urine. The presence of cytotoxic or cytostatic agents, cell culture additives and mitogenic materials in supernatant fluids can influence many bioassay procedures. Serum or plasma can cause matrix effects in many assays, and it is very important to validate methods for appropriate use with particular biological fluids.

If blood levels of cytokines are to be assessed, it is essential to ensure that post-collection processes (e.g. coagulation) do not cause cell activation and release of cytokines, and a possible misinterpretation of results. In most cases, it is best to use plasma as the assay material, thus avoiding coagulation altogether. However, several anticoagulants (e.g. EDTA or citrate, which chelate divalent ions like calcium) can interfere with cytokine bioassays. In our experience, a low concentration (2IU/ml) of preservative-free heparin is the best anticoagulant for most cytokine assays. Plasma or serum should be separated from blood cells as soon as possible and stored at $\leq-20°C$ until assayed.

A frequent problem with tissue fluids is the presence of soluble receptors, cytokine autoantibodies or other binding proteins that may mask activity. Thus, extraction of the cytokine may be necessary before assessment of cytokine activity. Some biological samples, e.g. plasma, may require special treatment prior to detection of certain cytokines by bioassay – heat treatment (56°C for 30 min) for IL-6, and acid activation (0.12M HCl for 30 min) for TGFβ.

STANDARDIZATION AND STATISTICAL EVALUATION OF CYTOKINE ASSAYS

The advent of recombinant DNA technology has enabled the identification, cloning and production of cytokines to be rapid and less complex. There are now many ways to produce cytokines using different expression systems (such as *E. coli*, yeast, and chinese hamster ovary, CHO, cells) for production of protein, or different methods to refold and stabilize the protein. This has led to the availability of many individual cytokines from different manufacturers, with each product possessing a distinct but different biological specific activity even when produced using the same source (e.g. *E. coli*). As a result, it is virtually impossible to calibrate correctly bioassays in 'mass' units as 1ng protein from one manufacturer can be quite different in biological potency to 1ng protein from another. Calibration in terms such as the ED_{50}, or '50% maximum proliferation', is also not suitable as it can vary considerably between laboratories, different bioassay systems for the same cytokine and even between experiments carried out in the same laboratories by the same methods but at different times. Some assays are more sensitive to the activity of a cytokine than others (particularly when the cytokine has pleiotropic activity), and thus many different bioassay systems may be used for its measurement. It is therefore necessary to have a single standard unit defined by an ampoule content and one that is assay independent, i.e. an ampoule of WHO International Standard for Interleukin 2 (IL-2) contains, by definition, 100 International Units of IL-2 regardless of the bioassay used (e.g. CTLL-2 cell line assay, or T cell mitogenesis assay).

As with all assays, it is essential that cytokine measurements are carefully and correctly standardized. The best approach for most systems is to use an arbitrary unitage directly related to that of a standard preparation. A range of such preparations for different cytokines – WHO International Standards and WHO Reference Reagents – is available from the NIBSC (Table 4.5). The biological potency unit assigned to ampoules of WHO Standards are purely arbitrary and can be used in any bioassay in any laboratory on successive occasions to produce comparable results.

Table 4.5 – The current list of available cytokine standards and their status.

Preparation	Product code	Status	Depository
IL-1α rDNA	86/632	IS	NIBSC
IL-1β rDNA	86/680	IS	NIBSC
IL-1 soluble receptor type 1 rDNA	96/616	IR	NIBSC
IL-2 cell line-derived	86/504	IS	NIBSC
IL-2 rDNA	86/564		NIBSC
IL-3 rDNA	91/510	IS	NIBSC
IL-4 rDNA	88/656	IS	NIBSC
IL-5 rDNA	90/586	RR	NIBSC
IL-6 rDNA	89/548	IS	NIBSC
IL-7 rDNA	90/530	RR	NIBSC
IL-8 rDNA	89/520	RR	NIBSC
IL-9 rDNA	91/678	RR	NIBSC
IL-10 rDNA	92/516	IR	NIBSC
IL-11 rDNA	92/788	RR	NIBSC
IL-12 rDNA	95/544	RR	NIBSC
IL-13 rDNA	94/622	RR	NIBSC
IL-15 rDNA	95/554	RR	NIBSC
G-CSF rDNA	88/502	IS	NIBSC
GM-CSF rDNA	88/646	IS	NIBSC
M-CSF rDNA	89/512	IS	NIBSC
Flt 3 ligand rDNA	96/682	IR	NIBSC
Onco M	93/564	RR	NIBSC
SCF rDNA	91/682	IR	NIBSC
LIF rDNA	93/562	RR	NIBSC
TGFβ$_1$ rDNA	89/514	IR	NIBSC
TGFβ$_1$ (natural bovine)	89/516		NIBSC
TGFβ$_2$ rDNA	90/696	IR	NIBSC
IFNα leukocyte	69/19	IS	NIBSC
IFNβ fibroblast	Gb23–902–531	IS	NIAID
IFNγ rDNA	GxgO1–902–535	IS	NIAID
TNFα rDNA	87/650	IS	NIBSC
TNFβ rDNA	87/640	RR	NIBSC
MCP-1 rDNA	92/794	IR	NIBSC
MCP-2 rDNA	96/594	IR	NIBSC
MIP-1α rDNA	92/518	IR	NIBSC
MIP-1β rDNA	96/588	IR	NIBSC
RANTES rDNA	92/520	IR	NIBSC
GRO/MGSA rDNA	92/722	IR	NIBSC
Bone morphogenetic protein-2	93/574	IR	NIBSC

[IS=International Standard: RR=WHO Reference Reagent: IR=Interim Reference Reagent: NIBSC=National Institute for Biological Standards and Control (UK): NIAID=National Institute for Allergy and Infectious Diseases (US).]

It is also essential that bioassay data are analysed correctly and are statistically evaluated. The WHO Standards are intended to be used as the primary calibrants for assays of biological potency and should be used to calibrate in-house standards. The most appropriate method to estimate biological activity using a reference standard is to use the parallel line approach. This involves the production of dose–response curves by a dilution series of both calibrant and unknown. It is important that at least four points of the series lie on the linear portion of the standard curve. The parallel portions of these curves are then used to measure the displacement of unknowns from the standard, which is proportional to the biologically active cytokine content of the samples. Basically, the displacement of the two curves is an indication of the relative potency of the two preparations from which the actual potency of the unknown can be derived. These curves should be parallel if the molecule responsible for the activity in samples and standards is the same. Alternatively, an approximate estimate of activity can be made by taking two or three points from the titration curve and reading these from the standard curve. To derive a potency for cytokine products intended for therapeutic use, a particularly careful assay design and a thorough statistical evaluation are essential.

Standardization of immunoassays for cytokines is made problematical largely by the possible microheterogeneity in cytokine structure (see above). In many cases, it is virtually impossible to standardize such methods in a way that allows a valid comparison between different assays and possibly different preparations of a cytokine. However, the need to standardize and calibrate cytokine immunoassays has been realised for some time and was the subject of a meeting held at NIBSC in November 1996. Representatives of immunoassay kit manufacturers, therapeutic product manufacturers and researchers were present. The data from WHO international collaborative studies presented at the meeting clearly showed that the use of a single standard drastically reduces interassay and interlaboratory variations. Although variation between different kits is still apparent, this is perhaps due to the unique recognition profile of individual antibody pairs and cannot be overcome. Therefore, it was decided by a majority view that WHO cytokine standards (initially intended only for assessment of potency in bioassays) should be used to calibrate immunoassay kit standards. Therefore, an active programme is ongoing to assess the suitability of cytokine potency standards not yet tested by international collaborative study to ensure that they can serve the dual purpose of being both a potency as well as an immunoassay standard. For the purpose of calibrating immunoassays, it was decided that mass could be used as the primary measure for estimating levels of cytokines.

CONCLUSIONS

Assessment of cytokine levels has not only contributed significantly to the understanding of cytokine biology and biochemistry, but also has provided insights about the involvement of cytokines in physiological and pathological processes. However, inappropriate assay choice or design can lead to confusion or even erroneous conclusions. Only if well-characterized and well-validated methods are used, and if the results are carefully analysed, can unambiguous information be obtained. Often it is necessary to use more than one assay system to confirm cytokine involvement in a particular process, and this situation is likely to become even more complex as the range of identified cytokines increases and as new procedures for cytokine detection and measurement are developed.

SELECTED READING FOR MORE DETAILED INFORMATION

An important paper describing a novel assay using transfected cells:
Abe M, Harpel JG, Metz DN et al. An assay for transforming growth factor-β using cells transfected with a plasminogen activator inhibitor-1 promoter luciferase construct. *Annals of Biochemistry* 1994; **216**: 276–282

Because preferential recognition may occur, this paper emphasizes the importance of the proper characterization of antibodies used in immunoassays for estimating cytokines:
Bird C, Wadhwa M, Thorpe R. Development of immunoassays for human IL-3 and IL-4 some of which discriminate between different recombinant DNA derived molecules. *Cytokine* 1991; **3**: 562–567

Provides details on the correct procedures for parallel line assays:
British Pharmacopoeia. Biological assays and tests, 1993, Appendix XIV, A164.

Both papers describe assay protocols for estimating cytokine production at the level of the single cell:
Labalette-Houache M, Torpier G, Capron A, Dessaint JP. Improved permeabilisation procedure for flow cytometric detection of internal antigens. Analysis of Interleukin-2 production. *Journal of Immunological Methods* 1991; **138**: 143–153

Lewis CE, Campbell A. Visualising the production of cytokines and their receptors by single human cells. In Balkwill FR (ed.). Cytokines: a practical approach, 2nd edn. Oxford: IRL 1995, pp 339–356

This paper emphasizes the importance of bioassays in the development and quality control of cytokines and other biological products:
Mire-Sluis AR, Gaines-Das RE, Gerrard T et al. Biological assays; Their role in the development and quality control of biological medicinal products. *Biologicals* 1996; **24**: 351–361

This paper highlights the importance of biological units, and illustrates the different specific activity of materials produced in identical expression systems:
Mire-Sluis AR, Gaines-Das R, Thorpe R. Implications for the assay and biological properties of interleukin-4: results of a WHO International Collaborative Study. *Journal of Immunological Methods* 1996; **194**: 13–25

This paper provides detailed information about the KIRA assay:
Sadick MD, Sliwkowski MX, Nuijens A et al. Analysis of heregulin-induced ErbB2 phosphorylation with a high-throughput kinase receptor activation enzyme-linked immunosorbant assay. *Annals of Biochemistry* 1996; **235**: 207–214

This paper provides protocols for the identification, using histochemistry, of cells involved in cytokine production:
Sander B, Andersson J, Andersson U. Assessment of cytokines by immunofluorescence and the paraformaldehyde-saponin procedure. *Immunological Reviews* 1991; **119**: 65–93

This paper describes a carefully characterized immunoassay validated for use with biological fluids:
Thorpe R, Wadhwa M, Gearing AJH et al. Sensitive and specific immunoradiometric assays for human interleukin-1 alpha. *Lymphokine Research* 1988; **7**: 119–127

This paper describes protein synthesis and cytokine mRNA expression:
Wadhwa M, Dilger P, Meager A et al. IL-4 and TNF mediated proliferation of the human megakaryocytic line M-07e is regulated by induced autocrine production of GM-CSF. *Cytokine* 1996; **8**: 900–909

These papers provide assay protocols for various cytokine assays:
Wadhwa M, Thorpe R, Bird CR, Gearing AJH. Production of polyclonal and monoclonal antibodies to human granulocyte colony-stimulating factor (G-CSF) and development of immunoassays. *Journal of Immunological Methods* 1990; **128**: 211–217

Wadhwa M, Bird C, Page L et al. Quantitative biological assays for individual cytokines. In Balkwill FR (ed.). Cytokines. a practical approach, 2nd edn. Oxford: IRL 1995, pp. 357–392

Several additional chemokines have recently been identified, and the following paper provides an up-to-date review of some their properties:
Luster AD. Chemotactic cytokines that mediate inflammation. *New England Journal of Medicine* 1998; **338**: 436–445

5

GROWTH FACTORS AND THEIR RECEPTORS IN HAEMOPOIESIS

C. J. Pallister and S. A. Marriott

SUMMARY

There has been an explosion of knowledge recently about cytokines and cytokine receptors, and the roles they play in cellular growth, differentiation and function. Nowhere has this growth in knowledge been more marked than in the area of haemopoiesis and haemopoietic growth factors (HGFs). However, growth in knowledge has been accompanied by an apparently exponential growth in complexity. This chapter aims to provide an overview of the classification of the different HGFs and to define the roles they play in the regulation of haemopoiesis. It does not pretend to be an authoritative or complete review: the emphasis is on aiding understanding of current knowledge and highlighting areas of ignorance in this important area of haematology.

HAEMOPOIETIC GROWTH FACTORS

Under normal physiological conditions, the number of circulating blood cells is maintained in remarkably narrow limits. Since all blood cells have a limited life span, a dynamic equilibrium must exist between cell loss due to senescence or normal function, and the synthesis and release of their replacements. Maintenance of this dynamic equilibrium requires a capacity for production of blood cells of astonishing fecundity coupled with exquisite responsiveness to the changing needs of the body for blood cells.

Our current understanding of the mechanisms that regulate haemopoiesis *in vivo* is far from complete. Advances in semi-solid cell culture techniques have led to the identification of a large family of glycoproteins required for optimal growth and differentiation of haemopoietic progenitor cells. The structure, synthesis and mode(s) of action of these haemopoietic growth factors (HGFs) have been studied intensively, and an overall picture of the complex regulatory mechanisms involved in the control of haemopoiesis is emerging.

The nomenclature of the HGFs is in dire need of revision to provide a more systematic and transparent method of classification (see Table 4.1 in chapter 4). The existing names are confusing and often misleading because they reflect the order of discovery or the first discovered function of the relevant factor. Many HGFs perform a variety of roles and act on a variety of cell types which may be quite different to those suggested by their name. For example, stem cell factor (SCF) has been shown to play important roles in spermatogenesis and melanogenesis, as well as in early haemopoiesis. This phenomenon of a single HGF having a large number of targets of activity is known as pleiotropy. Further, the action of given HGFs with specific targets commonly is duplicated by other HGFs, a phenomenon known as redundancy. The twin features of pleiotropy and redundancy are hallmarks of the function of HGFs.

In essence, the function of all cytokines is to transmit signals between sensor cells and effector cells. For example, when a requirement for erythrocyte production is sensed as tissue hypoxia by cells in the kidney, erythropoietin is secreted in the circulation and transported to the bone marrow, where it binds to specific receptors on erythroid precursors and stimulates erythropoiesis. This generalized pattern of sensor cells synthesizing and secreting cytokines in response to stimuli, followed by binding of the cytokine via specific surface receptors on effector cells holds true for all cytokine HGFs which influence blood cell production or function.

The purpose of this chapter is to review the properties and functions of the most important HGFs and their respective receptors. Although the HGFs are discussed individually, they exist *in vivo* as complex mixtures whose actions can be synergistic and/or antagonistic.

MOLECULAR GENETICS OF THE HGFS

Structure and expression of HGF genes

One of the most striking observations about HGF genes is their tendency to cluster in the genome. For example, the genes that encode IL-3, IL-4, IL-5, IL-9, IL-12β, IL-13 and GM-CSF are all located at 5q23–31. The M-CSF receptor gene also is located in this region. Deletion of this region is associated with a subtype of myelodysplastic syndrome (5q-syndrome), which is characterized by refractory macrocytic anaemia, thrombocytosis, splenomegaly and a low rate of progression to acute leukaemia. This arrangement, coupled with the similarity of gene structure, probably indicates evolution from a common ancestral gene.

If HGFs are to succeed in their major role as players in the haemopoietic orchestra, their local concentrations must be rapidly and finely adjustable. This requires that gene expression is closely regulated and that the clearance times of the elaborated proteins are short. Normally these requirements are readily met: resting or unstimulated cells do not synthesize detectable levels of HGF but are capable of rapidly initiating mRNA transcription following stimulation. The circulating half-life of most HGFs is <15 min.

Regulation of HGF gene expression is at the level of mRNA transcription. In common with other genes, HGF gene expression is governed by upstream promoter sequences which, via binding of various nuclear proteins, either inhibit or promote transcriptional activity. It is thought that external cellular stimulation, for example by bacterial lipopolysaccharide, triggers an internal signalling cascade which causes the expulsion of inhibitory nuclear proteins from the promoter sites and facilitates the binding of stimulatory proteins. The result is a rapid and substantial activation of mRNA transcription.

Stability of transcribed mRNA also appears to play an important role in the regulation of HGF gene expression. Sequence analysis of HGF mRNA has revealed a downstream structural motif consisting of multiple copies of the sequence AUUUA, which acts as a target for ribonuclease-mediated digestion. Thus, in resting cells, HGF mRNA is short-lived and does not result in translation of protein. Stimulation of the cell, however, is associated with temporary inhibition of the ribonuclease, thereby allowing prolonged survival of transcribed mRNA and promotion of translation and secretion of mature protein.

Structural classification of the HGFs

One of the most useful classification systems for the HGFs utilizes their three-dimensional conformation as its basis. The overall shape of a protein molecule is determined by the C^α—C and C^α—N bonding arrangements that it contains which, in turn, is determined by the amino acid sequence. A small number of structural motifs recur in proteins, namely the α helix and β-conformations such as pleated sheets, trefoil, jellyroll, meander and cysteine knot. In the right-handed α-helix composed of L-amino acids, the backbone of the polypeptide chain is arranged in a helix with 3.6 amino acids per turn. The degree of rotation for all C^α—C bonds is –47° while that of all C^α—N bonds is –57°. This results in a stable conformation because the C=O group and the N—H group of the peptide bond are orientated in such a way that the formation of a network of intrachain hydrogen bonding is promoted. Further, the α-helix forces the R groups of the amino acids to point outwards, thereby minimizing destabilizing interactions. The β-conformations are characterized by extended sheet-like folding of the polypeptide chain and are stabilized by perpendicular intrachain hydrogen bonds. The sheets may run in the same direction (parallel) or in opposite directions (antiparallel). A single protein molecule commonly contains more than one of these motifs.

Using the structural classification system, four groups of HGFs are recognized, which are characterized by the following features:

- group 1: antiparallel 4-helical bundle structures (e.g. GM-CSF);

- group 2: long chain β sheet structures (e.g. TNF);

- group 3: short chain /β structures (e.g. EGF); and

- group 4: mosaic structures (e.g. IL-12).

Group 1 HGFs

The group 1 HGFs are members of the largest family of cytokines and are characterized by the presence of an antiparallel 4-helical bundle structure. This group can be divided into two groups according to the length of the α-helices:

- short chain types are characterized by α helices of about 15 amino acids, a relatively large skew of about 35° between the AD and BC helix pairs and their flattened elliptical shape. Examples of this group of HGFs include IL-2, IL-3, IL-4, IL-5, IL-7, IL-9, IL-13, GM-CSF, M-CSF, SCF and IFNγ; and

- long chain types are characterized by α helices of about 25 amino acids, a relatively small skew of about 18° and their elongated cylinder shape. Examples of this group of HGFs include IL-6, IL-12, IL-10, IL-11, Epo, G-CSF and LIF.

Most of the group 1 HGFs bind to receptors that contain a 200 amino acid binding region, called the haemopoietin domain, and which have no intrinsic tyrosine kinase activity. The few exceptions to this rule include IL-10 and IFNγ which bind to interferon receptor-like proteins, and M-CSF and SCF which bind to immunoglobulin domains of class III tyrosine kinase receptors (see below). The binding domains of the interferon receptor-like proteins and the immunoglobulin domains of class III tyrosine kinase receptors are structurally related to the haemopoietin binding domain.

Most of the group 1 HGFs require heterodimeric receptors for high-affinity binding or to exert their biological effects. These receptors are differentiated by their unique, ligand-binding α-chains, but typically they share a common chain. For example, IL-2, IL-4, IL-7, IL-9 and IL-13 all share a common γ-chain; IL-3, GM-CSF and IL-5 share a common β_c chain and IL-6, LIF and IL-11 share a common chain designated gp130.

Group 2 HGFs

The group 2 HGFs can be divided into three families, each characterized by their own structural stigmata:

- members of the tumour necrosis factor family exist as cell surface-associated symmetric homotrimers and carry a characteristic β-jelly roll conformation. This family of HGFs bind to type I or II members of the TNF receptor family;

- IL-1 and fibroblast growth factor families display complex β-trefoil (clover leaf-shaped) conformations. These HGFs bind to receptors that carry extracellular immunoglobulin domain repeat regions; and

- PDGF and TGFβ have cystine knots composed of four twisted antiparallel β-sheets interlinked by disulphide bridges. PDGF-like HGFs bind to class III tyrosine kinase receptors while TGFβ-like HGFs bind to specific receptors with serine/threonine kinase activity.

Group 3 HGFs

The group 3 cytokines can be divided into three families:

- the epidermal growth factor (EGF) family, which are synthesized as transmembrane precursor molecules with the active EGF domain(s) in the extracellular region. Mature epidermal growth factor is a 53 residue polypeptide characterized by two antiparallel β-sheets connected by disulphide bonds to the joining loops. Other family members are larger molecules. Members of this family exert powerful mitogenic effects on a range of tissues but have no haemopoietic effect and so will not be considered further. EGF-related cytokines bind to class I tyrosine kinase receptors;

- the insulin-related family, characterized by three short-chain α-helices, is linked by three highly conserved disulphide bonds. Insulin-related HGFs bind to class II tyrosine kinase receptors; and

- the chemokine family, which adopts the conformation of an open-faced β-sandwich with a C-terminal α-helix and is characterized by the presence of four conserved cysteine residues. This group can be divided into two subgroups according to the amino acid sequence around the conserved cysteine residues (C-C or C-X-C). Examples of the former group include MCP-1, 2 and 3, MIP-1α and MIP-1β, while examples of the latter group include IL-8, MIP-2 and NAP-2. Chemokines bind to serpentine receptors which are coupled to G-proteins.

Group 4 HGFs

Some cytokines are characterized by mosaic structures of more than one of the above types. For example, neuregulins contain both an EGF and an immunoglobulin-like domain in their extracellular regions. IL-12 is a heterodimer with an α-chain typical of long-chain 4α helical bundles and the β-chain includes a haemopoietin domain.

HGF receptors

The biological action of a polypeptide ligand or cytokine is exerted through receptors expressed on the surface of the target cell. Ligand binding triggers a series of events that lead to the generation of cellular signalling mediated through intracellular protein kinase phosphorylation.

Cell surface receptor occupancy constitutes the 'first messenger' which emits one or more intracellular signals that alters the behaviour of the cell. The message is relayed across the cell membrane to influence events (generation of new intracellular signals through 'secondary messengers') in the cytosol and, eventually, in the nucleus. HGFs and their receptors form complex signalling networks that act as positive or negative regulators of cell proliferation and differentiation. Signalling pathways inside a cell are non-linear and form a network with multiple cross talking among the different pathways. Therefore, the ligand-binding domain of the receptor may not be the sole determinant of the cellular responses; a single receptor may couple to multiple signal transduction systems. Conversely, multiple receptors may couple to the same signal transduction pathway via common transducers or effectors.

The classification of the HGF receptors is more straightforward than for the cytokines themselves and is based on a combination of structural similarities and biochemical activity:

- haemopoietin receptors;

- receptor kinases;

- TNF receptors; and

- G-protein-coupled receptors.

Haemopoietin receptors

Members of the haemopoietin receptor family are integral membrane glycoproteins with their N-terminus outside the cell and a single membrane-spanning domain. Haemopoietin receptors exhibit a high degree of homology in their extracellular domains, including a 200 amino acid (D200) domain near the N-terminus region, a series of conserved hydrophilic and hydrophobic residues, a 60 amino acid domain which contains conserved cysteine residues that form disulphide bonds, and the characteristic motif with the consensus Trp-Ser-Xaa-Trp-Ser (WSXWS box) at the C-terminus. Although receptors in this family lack intrinsic tyrosine kinase activity, the cytoplasmic portion of the receptor associates with intracellular tyrosine kinases of the Janus kinase family (Jak-2).

The haemopoietin receptor family can be subdivided into three separate groups according to their subunit composition:

- group I includes single chain receptors that undergo homodimerization in response to ligand binding. Examples include the receptors for Epo, G-CSF and Tpo (thrombopoietin);

- group II receptors contain two different subunits, forming the high-affinity receptors via heterodimerization. Examples include the receptors for IL-3, IL-5, GM-CSF and IL-6; and

- group III includes high-affinity receptors composed of three different subunits. Examples include the receptors for IL-2, IL-4, IL-7, IL-9, IL-11, IL-15 and LIF.

Group I single chain receptors

Epo receptors are expressed on the surfaces of erythroblasts and erythroleukaemic cells. The receptor, which is glycosylated after synthesis, is of 507 amino acids. The extracellular domain binds Epo with high affinity, triggering homodimerization of the Epo-R and forming the high-affinity receptor required for signal induction. Although the cytoplasmic portion of the receptor does not contain a protein kinase domain, attachment of the Epo ligand induces protein tyrosine phosphorylation within the cell via the cytoplasmic protein tyrosine kinase Jak-2. On activation of Jak-2, a cluster of cellular proteins becomes phosphorylated. The phosphorylated tyrosine residues on the Epo-R complex serve as docking sites for proteins containing *src* homology 2 (SH-2) domains and the regulatory subunit of phosphatidylinositol-3-kinase (PI-3).

The G-CSF receptor, like Epo-R, consists of a single-chain receptor that traverses the membrane once, dividing the receptor into halves, namely the extracellular ligand-binding domain and a cytoplasmic portion that contains a proline-rich region involved in the binding of intracellular tyrosine kinases such as Jak-2. The N-terminal domain of G-CSF-R contains a 100 amino acid immunoglobulin-like sequence followed by the 200 amino acid haemopoietin, four conserved cysteine residues and the C-terminal WSXWS box. The 300 amino acid domain proximal to the transmembrane region is composed of three fibronectin type III-like sequences. The overall structure of the extracellular domain is homologous to that of the IL-6-R subunit gp130. The cytoplasmic domain has some homology to the IL-4-R.

Group II two different subunits receptors

The receptors for IL-3, IL-5 and GM-CSF each consist of a cytokine-specific α-subunit and a β-subunit common to all three. The α-subunits for the three receptors are ligand-specific but bind the ligand with low affinity. High-affinity receptors are formed when the ligand-specific α-subunit dimerizes with the common β-subunit. The β-subunit cannot bind ligand. Neither α nor β subunits have intrinsic kinase activity, but both units are required for signalling. The extracellular domains of the α-subunits contain common features of the haemopoietin family that include the four conserved cysteine residues and the WSXWS box motif near the transmembrane domain. As a consequence of the shared β-subunit, IL-3 and GM-CSF induce similar signals and their tyrosine phosphorylation patterns are almost identical. The distal region is also responsible for the major tyrosine phosphorylation and PI-3 kinase activation.

The α-subunits that form receptors for IL-3 are expressed on the surface of many cell types: IL-5-R α-subunits are found on eosinophils and basophils; GM-CSF-R α-subunits are expressed on haemopoietic progenitor cells, neutrophils, eosinophils and macrophages. The shared β-chain of the receptors IL-3, IL-5 and GM-CSF leads to competition for the binding of the respective HGFs to form the high-affinity receptors. Signalling requires the cytoplasmic domains from both the α- and β-chains and proliferative signalling through the cytoplasmic domain of the β-chain is localized to two short sequences (Arg456 to Phe487 and Val518 to Asp544) proximal to the transmembrane region. The C-terminal domain of the β-chain is responsible for tyrosine phosphorylation and activation of the MAP kinase pathway.

Jak-2 associates with the membrane proximal cytoplasmic domain of the β-chain. The kinase may activate directly cytoplasmic transcription factors of the STAT family.

The IL-6 receptor has two subunits: a ligand-binding chain and a non-ligand-binding domain signal transducer, gp130. Both chains contain the conserved cysteine residues and the WSXWS motif in their extracellular portions. The binding of ligand to the IL-6 receptor triggers association of the ligand binding subunit with the transducer receptor chain forming the high-affinity binding site resulting in signal transduction via gp130. gp130 has no IL-6 binding ability, and association of the IL-6 receptor and gp130 chain is necessary for signal transduction. Once the ligand has bound to the IL-6 receptor chain and the initial heterodimerization of the gp130 chain to the IL-6 chain has occurred, another gp130 chain undergoes homodimerization via disulphide links to the gp130 unit already attached. This structure composed of an IL-6 receptor chain and two gp130 subunits associates with a tyrosine kinase and tyrosine phosphorylation of gp130 takes place.

The gp130 subunit is not unique to the IL-6 receptor; it is required in the formation of several other receptors (e.g. LIF and IL-11) and is essential for signal transduction, thereby acting as a common signal transducer.

Group III three subunit receptors

Group III receptors contain three distinct subunits to make up the high-affinity functional receptor capable of signal transduction. The IL-2 receptor is formed when three different chains (α, β and γ) combine in response to ligand binding to the specific α-chain. The β- and γ-chains, which belong to the haemopoietin family, are required for the formation of the high-affinity receptor and also for signal transduction. Only when all three subunits come together can a signal be initiated. The γ-chain is not unique to the IL-2 receptor as it has been shown to form heterodimers with IL-4, IL-7, IL-9 and IL-15-specific chains and is therefore termed the γ-common subunit.

Receptor kinases

The members of this family of receptors, unlike the haemopoietin receptors, possess their own ligand-sensitive intrinsic kinase activity located within the cytoplasmic domain of the receptor. Not only is the signal transduced in this part of the receptor, but also the biochemical message is generated here. The first stage in signal transduction is the phosphorylation of the intrinsic kinase. The signal is then propagated by the phosphorylation of tyrosine, serine or threonine residues in cellular signal transduction pathway proteins. Activation of the signalling cascades normally is a consequence of the extracellular domain of the receptor binding its specific ligand. Several mutations have been described that result in a constitutive phosphorylation of the receptor and hence an unremitting activation of signal transduction pathways.

Kinase receptors are divided into three main domains:

- a large, extracellular ligand-binding domain that interacts with the polypeptide ligand;

- a short, hydrophobic transmembrane domain that anchors the receptor into the membrane; and

- a cytoplasmic domain capable of generating a signal that results in a pleiotropic response. The cytoplasmic portion can be further subdivided into the juxtamembrane domain, tyrosine kinase domain and the carboxy-terminal tail (C-tail).

Receptors normally exist as a single polypeptide chain in the unoccupied state and dimerise upon interaction with their cognate ligand. This homodimerization is an important step in activation of the majority of tyrosine kinase receptors.

The classification of the receptor tyrosine kinases into various subclasses is based on sequence similarity and their distinct structural characteristics:

- subclass I receptors are monomeric in structure and posses two cysteine-rich sequences in the extracellular domain. The cytoplasmic tyrosine kinase domain is uninterrupted in this class of receptors. Examples of this subclass include the receptors for EGF and *erbB*-2;

- subclass II receptors function as heterotetramers composed of two identical α- and two identical β-chains linked by disulphide bonds. The α-chains contain one cysteine-rich repeat domain each and form the ligand-binding domain. The α-chains are linked to the β-chains by disulphide bridges. It is the β-chains that traverse the membrane and contain the kinase domains (one per chain) in their cytoplasmic portions. The cleavage of the receptor precursor from a single gene product is responsible for the α- and β-chains. Examples of this receptor subclass include the receptors for insulin and insulin-like growth factor (IGF);

- subclass III receptors are distinctly different from the previous two subclasses. The extracellular domain lacks the cysteine repeat domains but contains another type of conserved repeat structure – five immunoglobulin-like domains. A hydrophilic insert of 68–90 amino acids divides the kinase domain in the cytoplasmic portion of the receptor which separates the ATP-binding and phosphotransferase kinase domains. Members of this receptor subclass include PDGF-R (A and B), M-CSF-R (*c-fms* product) SCF-R (*c-kit* product). Interestingly, *c-fms* is tandemly arrayed with the PDGF-R$_B$ gene while *c-kit* is similarly arranged in tandem with the PDGF-R$_A$ gene. This arrangement indicates duplication of an ancestral gene pair followed by independent mutation and divergence;

- subclass IV receptors of the fibroblast growth factor receptor (FGF-R) family contain a single membrane-spanning domain. The extracellular region is characterized by three consensus immunoglobulin-like domains and a short acid box domain located between Ig-1 and Ig-2. The cytoplasmic tyrosine kinase domain is divided in two almost equal portions by a short kinase insert of 14 amino acids. These receptors are expressed in multiple forms as a result of tissue-specific alternative splicing;

- the vascular endothelial growth factor receptors (VEGF-R), Flt-1 and KD-R form subclass V of the tyrosine kinase receptor family. The extracellular region contains seven immunoglobulin-like domains and the cytoplasmic tyrosine kinase is interrupted by a kinase insert. Flt-1 and KD-R share 30% sequence identity with M-CSF-R. Expression of these receptors appears to be restricted to endothelial cells;

- hepatocyte growth factor receptor (HGF-R, also known as scatter factor) is a heterodimeric receptor composed of an extracellular α-subunit linked by disulphide bridges to the membrane-spanning β-subunit. This factor forms subclass VI of the tyrosine kinase receptor family;

- subclass VII encompasses a family of neurotrophin receptors (TrkA, B and C) characterized by the presence of a tandemly repeated cysteine motif in the extracellular domain. Following ligand binding, Trk receptors homodimerize resulting in tyrosine kinase activation. Multiple forms of the Trk family members are expressed as a result of alternative splicing. A second class of neurotrophin receptors is widely expressed in both neuronal and non-neuronal tissues but carry no known enzymatic function;

- subclass VIII forms the largest family of tyrosine kinase receptors, the Eph-like receptors. The extracellular regions of these receptors contain an amino-terminal cysteine-rich domain followed by two fibronectin III domains, suggesting that these receptors may be involved in cell adhesion. The cytoplasmic tyrosine kinase domain is not divided. The nature of the ligands and function of the Eph-like receptors remain obscure; and

- a single member, the product of the *axl* gene, as yet populates subclass IX. This receptor is a 140 kDa protein related to the insulin and Eph-like receptor families. The extracellular region contains two amino-terminal immunoglobulin-like domains followed by two fibronectin III domains. The ligand(s) for Axl remain to be identified.

TNF receptors

The characteristic feature of the TNF receptor family is a repeated extracellular domain which contains six cysteine residues. TNF receptor family members include type I TNF-R (p60TNF-R, type B TNF-R), type II TNF-R (p80TNF-R, type A TNF-R), CD27, CD30, CD40 and FAS. Type I TNF-R and FAS also show considerable homology in their cytoplasmic domains, which are involved in the regulation of apoptotic signalling.

G-protein coupled receptors

G-protein-coupled receptors are characterized by their serpentine structure which traverses the cell membrane seven times. This class of receptors is extremely diverse and includes neurotransmitter, hormone, light and smell receptors as well as cytokine receptors. Examples of HGFs that bind to serpentine, G-protein-coupled receptors include MCP-1, 2 and 3, MIP-1α and β, IL-8, PF-4, MIP-2 and NAP-2. Two forms of the IL-8 receptor exist: IL-8R$_A$ and IL-8R$_B$, both of which bind IL-8 with high affinity and are expressed on neutrophils, monocytes, fibroblasts and lymphocytes. IL-8 also binds to a promiscuous chemokine receptor, which is expressed on human erythrocytes where it acts as a receptor for *Plasmodium vivax*. This receptor also binds other chemokines such as MCP-1 and RANTES and is thought to function as a regulator of inflammation by 'mopping up' excess circulating chemokines.

Regulation of blood cell growth, differentiation and function by HGFs and their receptors

Much of our current knowledge of the role of HGFs in the regulation of blood cell growth and differentiation has been derived from *in vitro* culture systems such as the CD34-enriched blast cell colony-forming (BCCF) assay and the high proliferative potential colony-forming cell (HPP-CFC) assay techniques. The results obtained have varied but certain common themes have emerged:

- the BCCF exists for much of the time in G$_0$ and in this state is independent of HGFs. These cells enter cycle randomly and are dependent on the presence of IL-3 for survival. Several HGFs, including IL-6, G-CSF, SCF and, in the murine system, IL-4, have been shown to act in concert with IL-3 to shorten G$_0$ and to improve the probability of successfully completing the cell cycle;

- the HPP-CFC requires a combination of IL-3 and GM-CSF to support their growth and development. SCF synergizes with these factors to promote cell growth. This assay correlates well with the capacity for haemopoietic reconstitution in the irradiated mouse;

- IL-3 is an effective supporter and promoter of CFU-GEMM colony formation *in vitro*. GM-CSF and SCF support IL-3 in this role. GM-CSF acts on more differentiated cells and preferentially supports development of neutrophil, eosinophil and macrophage colonies. There is some limited evidence that IL-3 acts as a growth factor for CD34+,CD7+ T lymphoid progenitor cells. IL-3 in addition to supporting development of multipotent colonies also promotes development of unilineage colonies such as erythroid, megakaryocyte and basophil colonies;

- CD3-,CD4-,CD8- (triple negative) thymocytes in the absence of mitogenic stimulation only respond to IL-2 when TNF is also present. Activated triple-negative thymocytes also respond to IL-4. CD3+,CD4-, CD8- thymocytes respond weakly to IL-7 and strongly to combinations of IL-2 and IL-1 or TNF. The addition of IL-1 or less convincingly IL-6 or TNF also augments the action of IL-7. The HGF requirements of CD4+,CD8+ thymocytes are currently poorly understood. CD4+,CD8- thymocytes respond to IL-2 and IL-7 singly or, more convincingly, when combined with IL-6. These cells are refractory to IL-4 alone but respond when this HGF is combined with IL-6. CD4-,CD8+ thymocytes respond best to IL-4 but also to a lesser degree to IL-2. The addition of IL-6 augments both of these responses. These cells are refractory to IL-7 alone but respond when this HGF is combined with IL-6;

- IL-7 is a growth factor for both pro- and pre-B lymphocytes but mature B lymphocytes are refractory to this HGF even following mitogenic stimulation. SCF synergizes with IL-7 as a promoter of early B lymphoid growth and development. IL-4 acts as an inhibitor of proliferation and promoter of differentiation of precursor B lymphocytes;

- production of late committed progenitors requires the presence of lineage-specific HGFs, e.g. G-CSF is required for optimal neutrophil production; M-CSF is required for macrophage development and survival; IL-5 is a required eosinophil growth factor; and the role of Epo in erythropoiesis has been well characterized. In other words, optimal production of mature cells requires the presence of both early and late-acting HGFs;

- resting T lymphocytes do not express IL-2-R and so are refractory to the action of this HGF. Triggering of the TCR complex leads to IL-2-R expression on the activated cell and production of IL-2 by various T lymphocyte subpopulations resulting in clonal autocrine growth of responding T lymphocytes. Synthesis of IL-1 and IL-6 by accessory cells is required to stimulate IL-2 production and to enhance responsiveness to IL-2 respectively. Activation of T lymphocytes can also be achieved via CD2 or CD28. The role of accessory cells as a source of IL-1 and IL-6 in CD28-mediated activation is similar but is not required for CD2-mediated activation. IL-4 has been shown to promote the growth of antigen-stimulated peripheral T lymphocytes while IL-7 stimulates mature splenic T lymphocytes in the presence of a co-mitogen. In both cases, part of the stimulation is achieved via IL-2 synthesis and IL-2-R expression but part appears to be the result of direct action by the HGF; and

- activation, proliferation of mature B lymphocytes and their differentiation into plasma cells is triggered by antigen stimulation and requires help from T lymphocytes. There is still considerable controversy surrounding the role that various HGFs play in this regard but IL-2, IL-4 and IL-5 (at least in mouse) probably all play a role in conjunction with antigenic stimulation. The activities of these HGFs are augmented by the presence of IL-1. IL-4 has been shown to promote secretion of IgM, IgG_1 and IgE antibodies; IL-5 to promote IgM, IgG_1 and IgA secretion; and IL-2 to promote secretion of IgM, IgA and all IgG subclasses. IFNγ inhibits secretion of IgG_1 and IgE. IL-6 is required for plasma cell production and growth.

CONCLUSIONS

There is compelling evidence that haemopoietic growth factors and receptors play a pivotal role in the regulation of haemopoiesis in health and disease. However, the complexity of the myriad actions, interactions and synergies is bewildering and it is almost beyond comprehension how such an apparently chaotic system can achieve the exquisitely fine control of blood cell production that characterizes haemopoietic health. Much remains to be elucidated and the challenge for the next decade is to characterize the system more completely. Such an achievement may well lead to therapeutic strategies which allow intervention when haemopoiesis is dysregulated in, for example, the leukaemias and myelodysplastic syndromes. Such a goal may seem a distant dream but the rate of accumulation of knowledge is accelerating greatly. Tomorrow may be closer than it seems!

ACKNOWLEDGEMENTS

The work of Dr SA Marriott is generously supported by a research grant from Amgen Ltd, Milton Rd Cambridge

SELECTED READING FOR MORE DETAILED INFORMATION

An authoritative but easy-to-read review of the biology of this important group of HGFs by a major author:
Metcalf D. The colony stimulating factors. *Cancer* 1990; **65**, 2185–2195

An excellent article describing the important but as yet poorly understood role of HGFs and their receptors in acute leukaemias. A greater understanding of the nature of leukaemic haemopoiesis and its regulation may well permit development of novel therapeutic strategies:
Lowenberg B, Touw IP. Hematopoietic growth factors and their receptors in acute leukemia. *Blood* 1993; **81**: 281–292

An example of early attempts to exploit the role of HGFs as primers of leukaemic blast cells to potentiate the cytotoxic activity of cytosine arabinoside. The responses of normal cells have been described in work previously published by these authors:
Smith MA, Singer CRJ, Pallister CJ, Smith JG. The effect of haemopoietic growth factors on the cell cycle of AML progenitors and their sensitivity to cytosine arabinoside *in vitro*. *British Journal of Haematology* 1995; **90**: 767–773

The cytokine homepage run by Horst Ibelgaufts at the University of Munich. It is a mine of useful information about cytokines and receptor-related information. The internet provides a particularly effective way of keeping up to date in this fast-moving area of biomedical science. The site is currently being reconstructed:
http://www.mb.uni-muenchen.de/groups/ibelgaufts/cytokines.html

Also run by Horst Ibelgaufts and accessible from the above web page, this site provides an authoritative guide to the jungle of synonyms, which have been used for various cytokines. If you are confused, start here!
http://www.mb.uni-muenchen.de/groups/ibelgaufts/alternatives.html

A commercially run web site (R+D Systems) providing up-to-date and authoritative reviews and updates. There is also a good deal of commercial information about sources and costs of cytokines for research use. Even if you are not interested in buying, this site is well worth a visit.
http://www.mdsystems.com

The cytokine web site at the University of Oxford's centre for molecular sciences is a mine of academic information. It is currently being reconstructed.
http: www.ocms.ox.ac.uk/cytweb

6

DIFFERENTIATION AND DEVELOPMENT OF B AND T CELLS

L. S. English

SUMMARY

B and T cell development in the bone marrow and thymus respectively are remarkably similar in that all the cells possess similar kinds of gene segments which are randomly assorted by almost identical antigen-independent mechanisms. However, there are some important differences in the two pathways. The random assortment of T cell genes in the thymus is meant to generate cells that bind to host MHC-foreign peptide. This inevitably results in the majority of T cells expressing receptors that either fail to bind to host MHC, and are therefore useless to the host, or which bind with high affinity to host MHC-self peptide and which would therefore be autoreactive. Selective processes in the thymus are designed to eliminate both these categories of cells leaving a small minority of T cells which exit the thymus and express receptors for host-MHC-foreign peptide. T cell development is, then, a totally antigen-independent phenomenon. In contrast, most B cells, irrrespective of their antigen specificity, undergo no selection in the bone marrow, but on being released into the periphery they depend for their survival on making contact and being activated by antigen – an antigen-dependent phenomenon.

INTRODUCTION

Haematopoietic stem cells and lymphocytic cells

There are some 10^{12} lymphocytes in an adult human. Around one-thousandth of these cells ($c.10^9$) die every day so there is a continual requirement for replacement for the individual to remain immunocompetent and to survive in a hostile environment. The bone marrow is the source of these cells, and fresh lymphocytes are produced by the proliferation of just a few haematopoietic stem cells which have the potential to produce any type of blood cell, i.e. they are pluripotential. These stem cells first appear in the yolk sac during the third week of embryo development, but at this stage no lymphocytes are produced. In the second month of development, blood cell formation transfers to the foetal liver and the first lymphocytes are seen in the blood. Shortly thereafter, the foetal spleen is involved, and by the fifth month the bone marrow has become the site of blood cell formation – a function that it maintains for the life of the individual. The liver and spleen cease production shortly before birth.

B and T cells

The pluripotential haematopoietic stem cells go through periods of self renewal in which they undergo cell division to generate more stem cells: at other times, the stem cells divide and differentiate, and through several generations develop to all the various types of blood cells – lymphocytes, monocyte/macrophages, granulocytes and erythrocytes. Progenitors for B and T lymphocytes arise from the stem cells in the bone marrow: B cell development continues in the bone marrow with the generation of mature B cells, which are then seeded to the periphery. The production of these cells continues in humans throughout life although with less efficiency as the individual ages and as the amount of functional haematopoietic tissue in the bone marrow decreases.

T cell progenitors, produced in the bone marrow, move to the thymus at a very early stage in their development where they mature into peripheral T cells. The rate of T cell production in the thymus is greatest during the early years of life: as early as the first year, thymic tissue involved in T cell development starts to shrink and continues to do so throughout life, being replaced by adipose tissue. However, the large pool of T cells in the periphery which are able to expand, together with a minority of T cells that may undergo extra-thymic maturation, appears to provide a sufficient number of T cells to maintain immunity throughout life: removal of the thymus, for example, late in life, does not result in any appreciable loss of T cell function.

Similarity in the developmental pathways of B and T cells

The development of B and T cells in the bone marrow and thymus respectively are remarkably similar. Both types of cells possess the same kinds of gene segments and the DNA rearrangement mechanisms are almost identical including expression of prereceptors. Both pathways are antigen-independent and involve deletion of potential autoreactive cells. However, there are also some distinguishing features in the two pathways:

- the great majority (≤95%) of potentially functional T cells are deleted in the thymus. This implies that a stringent selection process takes place at the immature T cell stage, and contrasts with B cell development, which allows most functional B cells to be released into the periphery where selection for survival subsequently takes place; and

- T cell receptors generated in the thymus maintain their specificity in the periphery, whereas most B cells have to modify their antigen specificity to survive.

B CELL DEVELOPMENT

B cell repertoire and chance meetings with antigen

The prime purpose of B cell development is to generate a sufficiently wide range of receptors by random mixing of the antibody genes to accomodate the vast array of antigens in the environment: millions of B cells representing this huge repertoire of antigen specificities are released continuously from the bone marrow to the periphery. Presumably, Nature's logic here is that, whatever antigen gains entry into the host, there will be sufficient B cells to respond, even though the majority will be useless. Most B cells die within a few days of release only to be replaced by more B cells, which will suffer the same fate. The process seems immensely wasteful but, since it works, it has to be considered efficient. The system almost guarantees that there will be enough B cells in this vast pool to express useful receptors which just happen to be there at the right time to respond when an antigen invades the host tissues. The major selection process for B cells is by antigen and takes place in the periphery.

Since a majority of the selected B cells may not be useful because they express low affinity for the antigen, Nature then imposes a second selection process which ensures that only the most useful (high affinity) cells survive as memory cells. However, it would appear that all cells have an equal chance at attaining that status since they all have the ability to modify their receptors, and those that achieve high affinity survive. The ways in which these objectives are achieved are explored below.

Bone marrow microenvironment and B cell development

Although it is possible to isolate small numbers of haematopoietic stem cells from the spleen, blood and thymus, the bone marrow appears to be the only site where development of all blood cell types occurs simultaneously. Non-lymphocytic stromal cells appear to be the major players in the development of blood cells: they appear crucial for blood cell development, and close contact through cell adhesion molecules (CAMs) between stromal cells and the developing cells seems essential for some of the developmental stages in the bone marrow. For example, progress of progenitor B cells to the pre-B cell stage occurs while B cells are in contact with stromal cells via various CAMs including VLA-4 (on B cells) interacting with VCAM-1 on stromal cells. Additionally, the interaction of kit receptor (CD117) on early B cells with stem cell factor (SCF) on stromal cells may provide a signal for early proliferation of B cells.

Stromal cells also secrete various cytokines that influence the progress of B cells through the various maturation stages. For example, interleukin 7 (IL-7) appears essential for the growth and progress of pre-B cells to immature B cells (see below), and IL-4 is necessary for the elaboration of IgM in pre-B cells. Receptors for IL-3 appear on progenitor B cells and persist through to the pre-B cell stage thus suggesting a function for this cytokine. Many other cytokines – IL-1, the colony-stimulating factors (G-CSF, GM-CSF and M-CSF), tumour necrosis factor (TNF), and transforming growth factor β (TGFβ) – may also induce changes in stromal cell activity to meet the demands for a particular cell lineage even though they may not necessarily be produced by stromal cells in the bone marrow.

Based on *in vitro* experiments, it appears that there is considerable heterogeneity in the stromal cell population, and that progress of B cells through the developmental stages may require more than one stromal cell type.

DNA rearrangements and stages in B cell development in the bone marrow

In the bone marrow, B cells go through a number of stages from progenitor stem cells to the immature B cell stage. The major developmentally programmed event that takes place during this period is the random rearrangement of the B cells' immunoglobulin genes resulting in the expression of IgM antigen receptors on the surface of B cells. This is followed by expression of IgD receptors expressing the same antigen specificity (the same light and heavy chain variable domains), and the cell moves to the periphery where it must make contact with antigen to survive. Before discussing this aspect in detail, it is appropriate to summarize the properties of human Ig genes and to explain how they rearrange to produce the huge repertoire of antigen specificities in B cells.

Chromosomal arrangement of immunoglobulin gene segments that encode the variable domain

At the 5' end of the Igh locus on chromosome 14 in humans, there is a cluster of about 50 functional variable segments (V_H), each of which encodes the amino acid sequence of framework regions (FRs) 1–3 and complementarity determining regions (CDRs) 1 and 2 – a total of about 95 amino acids (Fig. 6.1). Further downstream are up to 30 diversity segments (D) each of which encodes part of CDR3 (2–15 amino acids) and, towards the 3ó end of the Igh locus, is a third gene cluster consisting of six functional joining segments (J) which encode the remainder of CDR3 and FR4 (about 13 amino acids in light chains and 16–21 amino acids in heavy chains). Further downstream are the constant region genes beginning with IgM, followed by IgD, with the remaining Ig constant region genes at the 3' end of the IgH locus.

Loci for the light chain kappa (κ) and lambda (λ) are found on chromosomes 2 and 22 respectively. There are no D segments in light chain genes so these consist of V (about 30 λ and 40 κ functional segments) and J segments (4 l and 5 k functional segments) only. Each V segment encodes CDR1 and 2, part of CDR3 and FRs 1–3: each J segment encodes the remainder of CDR3 and FR4 (Fig. 6.1).

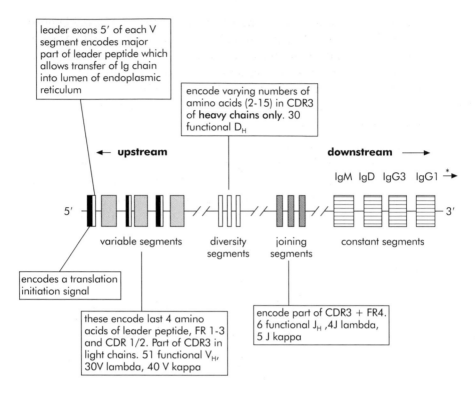

Figure 6.1 – Organization of germline Ig genes at the Igh locus (not to scale). The constant genes (represented by a single box) actually consist of many segments, each encoding a single domain. For example, there are four segments in the IgM constant gene encoding the CH1 to CH4 domains. There are extra segments encoding the IgM tailpiece (secreted IgM) or the transmembrane and cytoplasmic regions (membrane IgM). IgG has an extra segment encoding the hinge region. All the constant genes for each antibody class are not shown but they continue downstream from the IgG1 gene in the sequence IgA1-IgG2-IgG4-lgE-IgA2★. Light chain genes have V and J segments only with single constant segments of which there may be multiple copies. The arrangement of the λ and κ genes varies from that shown for the heavy chain genes.

Basic DNA rearrangement mechanism

Somatic recombination in a fairly random manner results in DNA rearrangement bringing together one of the many V segments, a D segment and a J segment in heavy chain genes. This provides a continuous message of VDJ as a complete heavy chain V gene, and a V segment with a J segment to form a VJ message as a complete light chain V gene. Thus, random mixing of these three segment pools can result in a large number of V genes to create a very large repertoire of antibody specificities.

During B cell maturation, the salient features of each step in this process include:

- somatic recombination of the heavy chain genes (Fig. 6.2) is followed by the joining of a D segment and a J segment which will thereby encode the CDR3-FR4 amino acid sequence of the antibody heavy chain. This rearrangement occurs on both chromosomes and many attempts to produce successful (productive) rearrangements are possible so long as there are D segments upstream and J segments downstream of the join; and

- in the second recombination event the cells attempt to join one of the 50 V segments with the rearranged DJ on one chromosome to form VDJ which is the complete variable gene. If this is productive, the cell undergoes transcription to produce a primary RNA transcript which is then spliced to produce a continuous RNA message (mRNA) for IgM

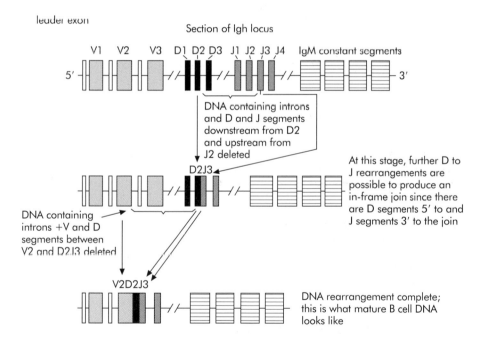

Figure 6.2 – Rearrangement of heavy chain genes in developing B cells. In the first somatic recombination, a D segment fuses with a J segment to form DJ, and this step is attempted on both chromosomes. If non-productive, further attempts can be made on the same chromosome as long as there are available D segments upstream from the joint and J segments downstream of it. In the second somatic recombination the DJ on one chromosome then fuses with a V segment to form a VDJ coding joint, which now encodes the whole V domain. A primary RNA transcript is produced and the intronic material and segments lying between the coding joint and the constant genes is spliced out producing a continuous RNA message (mRNA). The leader peptide is cleaved off the synthesized protein to give an IgM heavy chain.

heavy chains. IgM heavy chains are found in the cytoplasm with low levels of surface IgM heavy chain (see below). Proliferation of the B cell now takes place to produce many copies all of which carry the same VDJ arranged gene.

About 50% of all pro-B cells fail to make successful 'in frame' DNA rearrangements and die in the bone marrow by apoptosis. Each B cell has two chances to make a productive V-to-DJ rearrangement: if the rearrangement fails on the first chromosome by the production of an 'out of frame' sequence, then a second attempt cannot be made since, in producing a VDJ rearrangement, all the remaining D segments are deleted from the chromosome. However, the cell will attempt another rearrangement on the other chromosome and only if this fails will the cell be lost. A productive rearrangement on one or other of the parental chromosomes also leads to allelic exclusion since production of the IgM heavy chain signals a cessation of heavy chain rearrangements. Thus, the antibody product of each B cell only bears the allotypes derived from a single parent (Gm, Am and Km allotypes). Furthermore, since at this stage there is no light chain production, expression of IgM on the cell surface requires production of a special invariant surrogate light chain as the heavy chain cannot be expressed alone. This surrogate light chain is made up of two Ig-like proteins: one λ5, which is similar to a constant domain, and the other is structurally similar to a variable domain with an added N-terminal sequence, and is called the VpreB chain. This surrogate light chain complexes with the freshly produced IgM heavy chains to produce a cell surface pre-receptor IgM monomer, which appears with the other members of surface antibody receptors Igα and Igβ. It is thought that this receptor is some sort of signal for survival and also heralds a proliferative phase to produce B cell progeny all expressing the same pre-receptor IgM.

Following cell proliferation, light chain rearrangements begin and light chains are produced. Rearrangement is thought to occur at either light chain locus and, as for heavy chains, is attempted first on one chromosome and, if non-productive, on the second chromosome. However, since there are no D segments in light chain genes, there can be many attempts on either chromosome to produce a successful rearrangement so long as there are V segments remaining upstream of the non-productive VJ join and J segments remaining downstream of it.

If there are no productive rearrangements at one light chain locus then the other locus will attempt to produce a productive VJ rearrangement. The end result will be production of either κ or λ chains. Synthesis of surrogate light chains is now terminated and the κ or λ light chains pair with the IgM heavy chain and monomeric IgM is expressed on the surface of the cells. The cells dies if light chain rearrangements fail (Fig. 6.3).

Non-germline mechanisms produce more antibody diversity

During DNA rearrangement, additional variability (called junctional diversity) can be created in the final antibody products by imprecise joining at the V–J

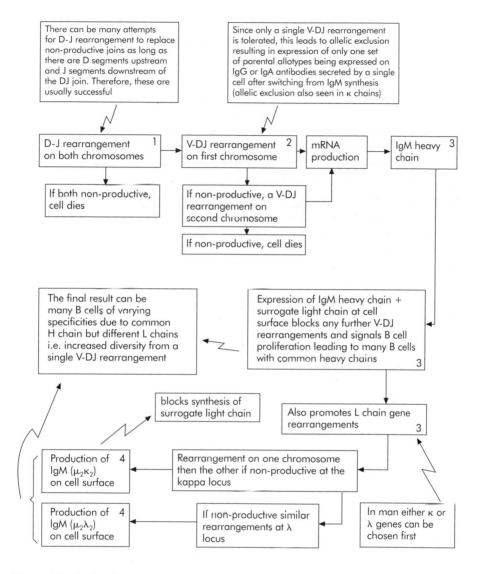

Figure 6.3 – Ordered rearrangements of Ig genes. Numbers indicate B cell stages in which events take place: [1] early pro-B; [2] late pro-B; [3] pre-B; and [4] immature B.

joints in light chain genes and at the D–J and V–DJ joints in heavy chain genes. Such rearrangements can completely alter the specificity of antibodies coded by productive joining of germline segments or could result in non-productive rearrangements. Additional diversity is generated by the action of the enzyme terminal deoxynucleotidyl transferase (TdT) which inserts extra nucleotides (the so-called N-nucleotides) at the $D-J_H$ and $V-DJ_H$ joints in heavy chain genes.

Germline and non-germline diversity

From the above review of the basic rearrangement mechanisms, and given that a set of V, D and J segments is inherited on each chromosome, it is possible to compare the contributions made to diversity by the germline and non-germline mechanisms. By randomly selecting V, D and J segments of heavy chain genes, and V and J segments of light chain genes, the potential total number of antibodies generated by germline mechanisms can be estimated. Given that there are 50 V segments, 30 D segments and 6 J sgements, there could be a total of 9000 heavy chains (50V × 30D × 6J), 120 λ chains (30V × 4J), and 200 κ chains (40V × 5J), giving a total potential number of antibodies of 2,880,000. The true number is likely to be considerably less as these estimates assume that all segments are used.

On the basis of this type of estimate it is therefore possible to conclude that many different antibodies can be created from each V segment since it has a choice of different D and/or J segments. However, these joins each result in a different CDR3 in the heavy or light chain so this creates the major proportion of diversity from one antibody to another. This contrasts with the number of CDR1 and CDR2 contact regions which are far fewer since they are carried on the germline V segments and their numbers equal the number of V segments in the genome.

Because of imprecision in the V–J, D–J and V–DJ joints, more diversity (termed non-germline) is created, all of which is at CDR3 sites and thus emphasizing the important contribution that this region makes to antibody specificity and diversity. In addition, there is a further mechanism – somatic hypermutation – that results in even more diversity. However, this is not operational unless B cells become activated and the immunoglobulin type switches from IgM to another class. In this process, the configuration of all CDRs is subject to change as B cells attempt to achieve high affinity status in their receptors (see below).

Control of rearrangement by flanking regions and recombination activating gene (RAG) enzymes

Immediately downstream from each V segment, upstream of each J segment and flanking both sides of each D segment, are strictly conserved heptamer sequences – usually CACAGTG or the inverted form CACTGTG – followed by a non-conserved spacer of 12 or 23 nucleotides (corresponding to one or two turns of the DNA helix), and then a nonamer sequence – usually ACAAAAACC or the inverted form GGTTTTTGT. When a coding joint is to be formed between two segments during rearrangement, the corresponding heptamers and nonamers are brought together and the intervening DNA between the segments is looped out. For two segments to join, the spacers between the signal sequences must be of the opposite type, e.g. D segments possess 12 base spacers and can join with either J or V segments which have 23 base spacers in the heavy chain. However, there is no direct joining between V and J in heavy chain genes since they both possess 23 base spacers (Fig. 6.4).

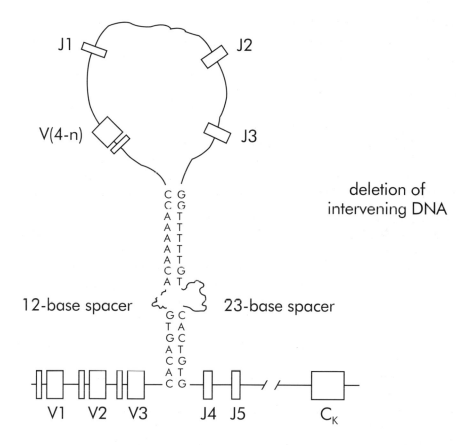

Figure 6.4 – Model for the joining of variable and joining segments in light chain genes during DNA rearrangement. Flanking regions are shown immediately downstream of the V3 (numbers are purely arbitrary) segment and upstream of J4 in an attempted joining of these two segments. The alignment of the conserved heptamers and nonamers and the 12- and 23-base spacers (opposite types) would promote fusion of the two segments under the control of RAG enzymes leading to deletion of all intervening DNA, including the signal sequences and the formation of a VJ coding joint. If this rearrangement was out-of-frame, a further rearrangement could occur involving the V segments upstream of the joint and J5. In some instances, when the V and J segments are in opposite orientation, a more complex DNA looping occurs (not shown).

Once the two segments are brought together by this arrangement, it is believed the actual joining is controlled by recombination activating genes (*RAG-1* and *RAG-2*). The previously looped-out section of DNA carrying intervening segments and intronic material is now excized as circular DNA and is destroyed. As expected, the RAG enzymes and TdT are only active during the B cell stages in which rearrangement occurs, i.e. from the early pro-B cell stages to the pre-B cell stages (see below).

DNA rearrangement steps and B cell development

While the schema outlined here is greatly simplified, each of the rearrangements discussed above is programmed to take place in a sequential manner during the various B cell stages (Fig. 6.5). In the first detectable stage of B cell development

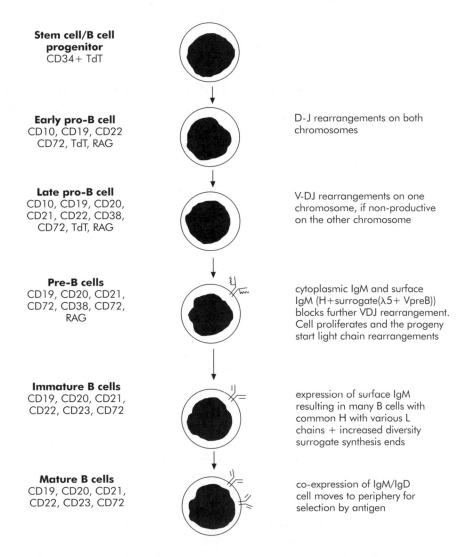

Stem cell/B cell progenitor
CD34+ TdT

Early pro-B cell
CD10, CD19, CD22
CD72, TdT, RAG

D-J rearrangements on both chromosomes

Late pro-B cell
CD10, CD19, CD20,
CD21, CD22, CD38,
CD72, TdT, RAG

V-DJ rearrangements on one chromosome, if non-productive on the other chromosome

Pre-B cells
CD19, CD20, CD21,
CD72, CD38, CD72,
RAG

cytoplasmic IgM and surface IgM (H+surrogate(λ5+ VpreB)) blocks further VDJ rearrangement. Cell proliferates and the progeny start light chain rearrangements

Immature B cells
CD19, CD20, CD21,
CD22, CD23, CD72

expression of surface IgM resulting in many B cells with common H with various L chains + increased diversity surrogate synthesis ends

Mature B cells
CD19, CD20, CD21,
CD22, CD23, CD72

co-expression of IgM/IgD cell moves to periphery for selection by antigen

Figure 6.5 – B cell development stages in the bone marrow. The principal activities and phenotypes of the cells are shown at each stage of development. B cells from all stages are thought to express the activation marker CD45R and MHC class ll. There is some confusion about what markers are present at each stage and those shown are not intended to represent all possible markers. TdT and RAG are intracellular enzymes. CD40 is thought to appear on the pro-B cell and to persist through to maturity.

– early pro-B cells – the D–J rearrangement takes place at the Igh locus on both chromosomes and the cells progress to the late pro-B cell stage. V–DJ rearrangement then takes place to produce IgM heavy chains and the cells are now recognized as being in the pre-B cell stage. The IgM heavy chains are expressed on the cell surface as pre-receptor IgM along with surrogate light chains (see above). Proliferation of pre-B cells initiates light chain gene rearrangements which, if successful, result in the production of light chains and the cell surface expression of IgM heavy chains covalently linked to either κ or λ chains. This proliferation of pre-B cells yields immature B cells.

During development and maturation of the B cell line there is an important connection between the production of a single in-frame VDJ rearrangement and expansion of the cell clone. The subsequent rearrangement of the light chain genes in these progeny results in many different light chain gene sequences, i.e. many different light chains, in cells all of which are producing the identical heavy chain. Thus, this proliferative step leads to considerable diversity in antibody products with the pairing of the diverse light chains with one heavy chain. This clever manoeuvre produces a variety of antigen specificities from a single VDJ rearrangement, thus increasing the probability that some of the B cell progeny will make contact with antigen in the periphery and thereby survive.

Mature B cell and expression of IgM and IgD

Before immature B cells leave the bone marrow, in addition to IgM they acquire surface IgD receptor molecules and become mature B cells. To produce both IgM and IgD receptors, B cells produce an extended primary RNA transcript, which includes the VDJ (encoding the antibody specificity) and, further downstream, the IgM constant message followed by the IgD constant message. Molecules of mRNA molecules are then constructed by alternative splicing-out of either the IgM or IgD constant message resulting in mRNAs for IgM and IgD heavy chains.

Removal or inactivation of potentially autoreactive B cells

Apoptosis ensures that cells that develop receptors recognizing self-antigens in the bone marrow are deleted. This is thought to happen when the antigens are widely distributed in the bone marrow. Examples of such antigens would be MHC molecules, CAMs and common CD (clusters of differentiation) molecules expressed on various cell types in close proximity to developing B cells. However, a minority of such B cells may be 'rescued' by further rearrangements of light chain genes resulting in receptors which may no longer be self-reactive and which transiently express two light chains on single B cells. This process is called receptor editing.

Other B cells expressing anti-self receptors for soluble antigens may develop and escape to the periphery, where they may come into contact with the antigens. Depending on the concentration of the antigen and the affinity of the receptors on B cells, the cells may die or become unresponsive (anergic) when they lose expression of IgM. Other self-reactive B cells never become activated since they cannot receive T cell help because T cell tolerance has been established.

Phenotypic changes in the developing B cell

From the preceding discussion, it is clear that pre-receptor IgM (IgM heavy chain with surrogate light chains) is expressed at the pre-B cell stage; IgM at the immature B cell stage, and finally IgM and IgD on mature B cells. In addition, other phenotypic changes occur during B cell maturation, possibly the most important of which is expression of a variety of CD molecules some of which are markers for particular developmental stages while others persist from the early stages of cell development right through to the mature B cell stage. Thus:

- MHC class II and CD45R (B220 – a signalling molecule) molecules are expressed on progenitor B cells and persist for the life of the cell;

- CD19, CD20, CD21, CD22 and CD72 appear at the pro-B cell stage and persist through to the memory B cell stage;

- CD10 is initially only expressed at the pro-B cell stage and reappears briefly when mature B cells become activated by antigen;

- CD23 – the low-affinity receptor for IgE – first appears at the immature B cell stage and then persists for the life of the cells;

- CD38 appears on the B cell surface in the early developmental stages but is lost at the pre-B cell stage. However, it reappears on B cells found in germinal centres and on plasma cells, and is also expressed on some T cells; and

- CD40 (a costimulator molecule) appears on pro-B cells and persists to the mature B cell.

Fig. 6.5 summarizes the above information and details the principal activities and phenotypic features of B cells during their development in the bone marrow.

Expression of Ig genes in early and adult life – CD5+ B cells

When animals are immunized with selected antigens during foetal life, their ability to respond appears to follow a consistent pattern, suggesting that B cell specificities develop in some programmed order. This implies that the use of V genes in foetal life is not random but follows a developmental pattern with the evidence indicating that the V_H segments nearest to the D segments are used first. For example, 80% of a selection of murine foetal or neonatal cells preferentially arranged one V segment, $V_H 7183$, situated at the 3' end of the V locus. Similarly, V_H Q52 in a similar position was also preferred.

It would therefore appear that foetal B cells rearrange a limited number of V genes to produce a limited repertoire of antibody specificities which contrasts with the range of antibodies representing the full repertoire of V genes produced in adult spleen. It is interesting to note that foetal B lineage cells do not express the enzyme TdT, which catalyses the primer-independent insertion of N-nucleotides during heavy chain gene rearrangement in neonatal and adult B lineage cells. As noted above, normal expression of this enzyme in adults leads to increased diversity of the antibody product.

In mouse, the earliest B cells that arise from the bone marrow are those expressing CD5 – a molecule also expressed by T cells. It is therefore possible that the observations discussed above refer, in large part, to CD5+ cells. These B cells have been classified as polyspecific as their receptors bind several different ligands with a preference for common bacterial antigens. Furthermore, their VDJ rearranged genes rarely undergo somatic hypermutation thus maintaining their germline configuration. CD5+ cells act in a T cell-independent manner and may have been conserved throughout evolution to provide protection against common bacterial pathogens encountered. In support of this hypothesis is the finding that CD5+ cells are located predominantly in the peritoneal and pleural cavities where they are ideally situated to encounter such antigens. In addition, they are capable of self-replication in the periphery which, since they are no longer produced in the bone marrow after early foetal life, ensures an adequate population. CD5+ cells are also prominent in many autoimmune diseases.

After birth, B cells developing in the bone marrow select a wider range of the V segments and possess TdT, thus being able to produce a wider range of antibody specificities. These cells, referred to as CD5- B-1a cells, are also self renewing in the tissues as the bone marrow finally switches to the production of adult B cells (B-2 B cells) which use the whole range of V segments. These undergo a number of non-germline methods of generating extra antibody diversity but are not self renewing since they are continually replaced by the bone marrow throughout life. Most of these cells have a short life span, apart from a minority which achieve memory cell status (see below).

B cells may survive in the periphery by encountering antigen

Although this section of the review focuses on B cell development in the bone marrow, it is important to appreciate that critical steps in the maturation of these cells occur after the cells encounter antigen in the periphery – indeed, only a small proportion of B cells survive for more than a few days in the circulation if they fail to contact antigen or fail to be selected by antigen during an immune response.

Naive B cells leave the bone marrow, enter the blood and then may migrate to lymphoid tissues. Here they may come in contact with antigen carrying the epitope which can be bound by the B cell antibody receptor. B cell proliferation will then occur if T cell help is available in T cell areas such as the paracortex of the lymph nodes. Some of the resulting B cell progeny will move to the follicles of B cell areas where they will come in contact with follicular dendritic cells (FDC), which carry antigen complexes known as iccosomes.

Sometime during this period of activation, the B cells, with T cell help through costimulation and secretion of cytokines, will class switch from IgM and IgD to express antibody receptors of some another class, e.g. IgG. The cells will then undergo an intensive round of somatic hypermutation in which apparently random mutations occur in the VDJ and VJ genes. Many of these mutations are localized in the CDR regions and result in modifications in receptor specificities of the cells. Those B cells that acquire higher affinity to the antigen will be 'rescued' from cell death, will become memory cells, join the recirculatory pool, and may become long-lived. Cells that fail to improve their originally low affinity for antigen, or lose their affinity, undergo apoptosis and die.

It has been estimated that many millions of B cells are produced daily by the bone marrow but these only replace an equal number which fail to survive in the periphery.

T CELL DEVELOPMENT

Requirement for thymic education in the development of T cells

Although there is much in common between the development of B and T cells, there is a crucial difference which reflects the manner by which these two populations recognize antigen. Unlike B cells that, through antibody receptors expressed on their surfaces, 'see' native or unprocessed antigen, T cells only 'see' linear peptides derived from antigens which are bound to self-MHC molecules expressed on various cells of the host.

It has been estimated that approximately equal numbers of B and T cells undergo productive rearrangements of the receptor genes resulting in a vast repertoire of antigen specificities. However, unlike B cells, where selection takes place in the periphery, the selection of useful T cells takes place in the thymus and the majority of cells deemed useless to the host are also eliminated there. The reason for this seems to be that only cells useful to the host have some affinity for self-MHC. Since T cell receptor (TCR) gene segments are to a large extent randomly assorted, the majority of productive rearrangements will not result in TCR with affinity for self but for allogeneic MHC products which are not present in the thymus in which rearrangement takes place – discussed further below. Such T cells cannot develop further and are eliminated in a screening process called *positive selection*.

A number of the positively selected T cells will have affinity for self-MHC when bound to self peptide rather than foreign peptide, and these potentially autoreactive cells cannot be allowed to escape to the periphery where they could cause damage to host tissues. Thus, a second selection process – *negative selection* – takes place, resulting in elimination of these cells and leaving a small minority of the total cells to enter the periphery as functionally mature T cells, which recognize only foreign peptide-self MHC.

These major steps in this process are summarized in Fig. 6.6, which describes schematically the fates of three progenitor cells: one cell fails to rearrange productively and undergoes apoptosis, whereas the other two succeed in forming productive rearrangements and proliferate to generate progeny that express TCRs on their surfaces. These cells then undergo positive selection in which most of the progeny will die if they fail to bind either MHC A or MHC B displayed by thymic epithelial cells. However, some of the progeny do bind MHC with sufficient affinity to survive, and these then undergo negative selection to remove potentially autoreactive T cells which would bind MHC-self peptide with medium-to-high affinity. These potentially autoreactive cells are eliminated, leaving the small proportion of T cells with low affinity for MHC-self peptide to migrate to the periphery as functional T cells where they can be activated by MHC-foreign peptide.

Actually, Fig. 6.6 greatly exaggerates the number of cells that mature successfully – only about 2% of the vast numbers of T cells generated in the thymus leave as functional T cells. Although there is thought to be a small number of T cells that develop outside the thymus, the process of T cell selection is in stark contrast with B cell development where selection of useful cells takes place principally in the periphery.

The thymus is essential for development of most T cells

In the early 1960s it was shown that the neonatally thymectomised mouse produced hardly any antibodies (because of no T cell help) and could not reject skin grafts (a T cell mediated immune reaction). More recently, it has been shown that the nude mouse (which normally lacks a thymus) produces no T cells unless a thymus is grafted when T cell production is restored. In man, patients with the rare immunodeficiency disease DiGeorge syndrome do not possess a thymus and also produce no T cells. Hence, the thymus appears essential for the development of T cells.

Thymic microenvironment

The thymus, situated in the upper thorax, just above the heart, consists of a number of lobules, each of which possess an outer cortex and an inner medulla. Rearrangement of T cell genes is mainly confined to pre-T cells in the cortex, and positive selection is thought to take place when the cells are in close contact with thymic epithelial cells expressing both MHC I and MHC II.

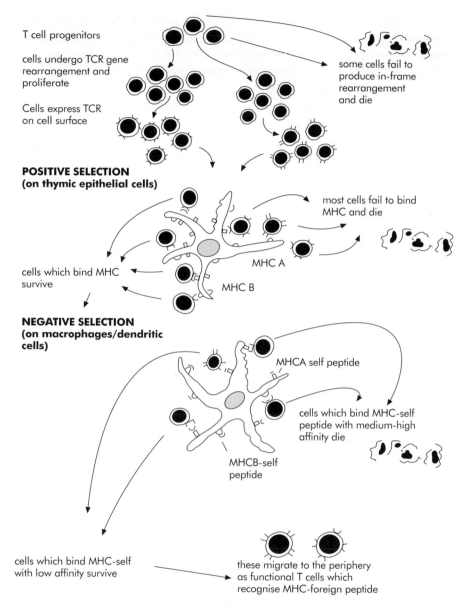

Figure 6.6 – Major events in T cell development.

Negative selection of T cells is thought to occur in the medulla or at the corti-co-medullary border where there is a predominance of macrophages and dendritic cells (professional antigen-presenting cells), again both expressing high levels of MHC I and II antigens.

The only cytokine that has been definitely implicated in T cell development is IL-7, which is thought to promote T cell gene rearrangement and proliferation of immature T cells. Experiments have demonstrated profound reductions in T cell numbers in the mutant mouse deficient in expression of IL-7R (the IL-7 receptor). Other cytokines such as IL-2 may be involved during the proliferative stages. As in B cell development, cell adhesion molecules are also crucial for proper T cell interactions and early T cell precursors have requirements for kit and SCF probably synthesized by thymic epithelial cells. Additionally, it is thought that CD28-B7 and CD40-CD40L co-stimulatory signals also play a major role in T cell development, although the exact contributions are still not known.

The T cell progenitor – bone marrow or thymus?

There is some dispute about whether thymopoiesis in the adult is dependent on a continuous supply of T progenitors from the bone marrow, or whether multipotential stem cells in the thymus sustain the supply of pre-T cells. Blood-borne progenitor cells have been detected, but this does not mean that they are destined for the thymus. In fact, some are destined for the gut (see below). It is known that in the post-natal human thymus, there are cells expressing the CD34+ stem cell marker which can develop to myeloid lines as well as T cells. Furthermore, there are cells in the adult mouse thymus that can develop to B cells, natural killer (NK) cells and dendritic cells, as well as T cells. These findings suggest that the thymus contains stem cells (albeit originally from the bone marrow) that may contribute to the supply of T cells and other cells especially in the adult thymus.

T cell development and bone marrow chimeras

It has already been noted that of the vast numbers of cells undergoing productive rearrangements of TCR genes, a large proportion fail positive selection because of their inability to show any binding affinity for host MHC. It was suggested above that some of these cells could bind to allogeneic MHC, and it follows that such cells could survive if they had been placed in a different MHC environment.

Experiments that support this idea have been done in the chimeric mouse (Fig. 6.7). This is an animal of, for example, strain B which has been neonatally thymectomized, irradiated and then reconstituted with bone marrow cells from a different strain (e.g. A). After a few weeks, T cells from strain B and B cells from strain A were injected in irradiated (A×B)F$_1$ mice, which were then immunized with antigen (sheep red blood cells: SRC). Do the A strain T cells that have developed in the B strain mouse provide help to A strain B cells? No anti-SRC antibodies were found in sera of the F$_1$ progeny (Fig. 6.7).

This result is perhaps surprising as it might be expected that A strain T cells would recognize the MHC-SRC peptide on A strain B cells, and thereby provide some help. This obviously did not happen. Rather, it appears that while the A strain T

A strain mouse

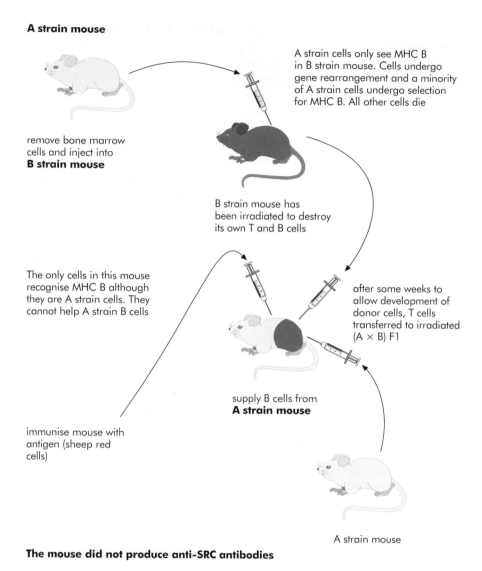

remove bone marrow cells and inject into
B strain mouse

A strain cells only see MHC B in B strain mouse. Cells undergo gene rearrangement and a minority of A strain cells undergo selection for MHC B. All other cells die

B strain mouse has been irradiated to destroy its own T and B cells

The only cells in this mouse recognise MHC B although they are A strain cells. They cannot help A strain B cells

after some weeks to allow development of donor cells, T cells transferred to irradiated (A × B) F1

immunise mouse with antigen (sheep red cells)

supply B cells from
A strain mouse

A strain mouse

The mouse did not produce anti-SRC antibodies

Figure 6.7 – Adaptive differentiation in bone marrow chimeras.

cells developed in a B strain thymus, only cells which recognized B strain MHC survived and matured. The majority of these cells would not have survived positive selection because their TCRs would not have affinity for MHC A. Similarly, A strain cells that developed TCRs for MHC A did not survive in the B strain mouse and hence no T cell help was forthcoming.

It thus seems that, irrespective of the source of T cells, random assortment of TCR genes will always result in cells that can successfully populate allogeneic members of that species: this is an interesting result with implications to bone marrow transplantation.

Two distinct lineages of T cells

As well as T cells that express the αβ pair of TCR chains (sometimes referred to as TCR2 receptors), there is a minor population of T cells which expresses different TCR chains composed of γ and δ pairs (TCR1). These cells express CD3 but are usually CD4- and CD8-, although a few cells do express CD8. Some express unusual specificities. For example, some human TCR1 T cells have been found to be broadly specific for the products of a number of MHC alleles, while others recognize a CD1 component. It is perhaps coincidental that CD1 binds and presents mycolic acid – a mycobacterial component – and some TCR1 cells have specificity for mycobacteria and their products. Yet other TCR1 cells recognize the MHC-like (TL) antigens in mouse but there are no reports of human cells recognizing the human equivalent.

TCR1 cells are the first T cells to appear in the foetal thymus. They also appear in the adult thymus, whereas others T cells appear to be thymus independent (therefore not MHC-restricted) and develop in epithelial tissues. TCR1 cells appear to be derived from the same stem cells as TCR2 cells but exhibit restricted antigen specificity using a small number of Vγ segments. Some human TCR1 clones have been shown to recognize classical MHC I and II associated, in some cases with known peptides.

TCR1 cells are predominantly found in epithelial tissues in all species examined and Vγ-restricted subsets in mouse appear to predominate in various tissues. For example, Vγ6- expressing cells are found predominantly in uterine epithelium, whereas Vγ7 and Vγ1 cells localize to intestinal epithelium.

The true function of TCR1 cells is not presently known although it appears that they may be the T cell equivalent of CD5+ B cells and may represent a primitive defence against a variety of common bacterial antigens.

TCR genes and rearrangement

T cell receptor genes

As noted above, T cells are divided in two major populations: the majority (TCR2) express receptors composed of a covalently linked α and β chains (αβ), while a minority population (TCR1) express a γδ combination (γδ).

The TCR genes (Fig. 6.8) are very similar to immunoglobulin genes with variable, diversity and joining segments:

- the α-chain genes have about 75 V segments, each with a leader exon: further downstream there is a cluster of about 60 J segments and a single constant gene;

Human TCR β chain locus (chromosome 7)

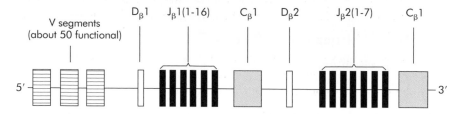

Human TCR α and δ chain locus (chromosome 14)

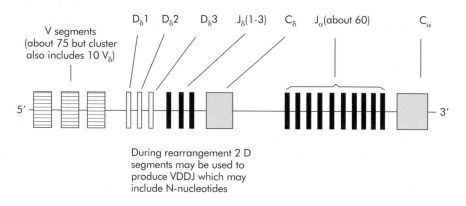

During rearrangement 2 D
segments may be used to
produce VDDJ which may
include N-nucleotides

Human TCR α chain locus (chromosome 7)

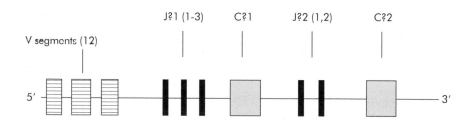

Figure 6.8 – Chromosomal arrangement of TCR genes (not to scale). Leader exons (not shown) are present upstream of each V segment.

- the β-chain locus is somewhat unconventional in that, downstream from the cluster of about 50 functional V segments, there are two distinct clusters each consisting of a single D segment with about six J segments. Yet further downstream is the constant gene;

- the δ-chain locus is most unusual in that it is situated between the V cluster and J cluster in the α-chain locus: this means that the δ-chain genes are deleted if there is an α-chain rearrangement. The V segments (<10) of the δ-chain locus appear to be situated in the V cluster: downstream there are three D and three J segments with a single constant gene; and

- the γ-chain locus probably has 10–20 V segments with a cluster of three J segments with one constant gene: further downstream is another cluster of two J segments with another constant gene.

The constant genes in all the TCR gene loci consist of segments encoding extracellular, hinge (where present), transmembrane and cytoplasmic regions of the TCR chains. As with antibody genes, the V segments encode CDR1 and 2, while CDR3s are constructed by rearrangement of either D and J segments, or V and J segments.

TCR rearrangement mechanisms

The rearrangement mechanisms for TCR genes are very similar to those discussed above for immunoglobulin genes. Thus, the signal sequences are the same and they are recognized by the same RAG enzymes. Additional diversity is generated at the joints by junctional diversity and insertion of N-nucleotides. However, in contrast with immunoglobulin light chain genes, N-nucleotides are also found at the V–J joints of α-chain genes. As with immunoglobulin genes, most of the diversity lies in the CDR3 nucleotide sequences of the rearranged TCR genes.

T cell development in the thymus

Stem cells and lineages

The earliest T cell precursor in the human thymus is thought to express CD34 (representative of bone marrow stem cells), CD44 and CD7, and probably contains cytoplasmic TdT and CD3 components (the ϵ and γ chains). Very early cells appear to express CD25 (IL-2αR) and these cells could be the progenitors of both TCR1 and TCR2 cells and, perhaps, thymic NK cells and thymic dendritic cells.

Early development of TCR1 cells

As little is known about human development, most knowledge on the early development of TCR1 cells deriving from studies on mouse. The first cells to appear in the murine foetus are $\gamma\delta$ T cells which have undergone rearrangement of the γ and δ chain genes. These cells are homogeneous since the most 5' J segment has been rearranged with the nearest V segment, Vγ5, in the absence of any junctional diversity. These cells predominantly migrate to the epidermis where, after a few days, they are replaced by cells which have rearranged the neighbouring V segment, Vγ6, but again with no added diversity. These are produced until birth and populate the epithelium of the reproductive tract. Both of these TCR1 cell populations appear to use the same rearranged δ-chain gene segments and so exhibit extremely restricted heterogeneity. Thus, it seems logical that these germline configurations may be important for defence against some common pathogens.

The Vγ6 cells are finally replaced after birth by a more heterogeneous population of TCR1 cells which have rearranged Vγ1, 2, 4, and 7, together with a number of δ-chain gene rearrangements, which includes a high degree of junctional diversity. There is increased diversity in the δ-chain gene since two D segments can be used in the same rearrangement, which also includes N-region diversity. A majority of these cells populates the intestinal epithelium. As indicated earlier, other TCR-1 cells may actually develop in the epithelium instead of the thymus.

Development of the TCR in TCR2 cells

In mouse, TCR2-expressing cells appear a few days after the first appearance of γδT cells. TCR gene rearrangements begin in double-negative (CD4-,CD8-), CD2, CD5 and CD7 cells starting with the β-chain gene: a DJ joint is formed followed by rearrangement with the V segment as for Ig heavy chain rearrangement. However, as noted above and shown in Fig. 6.8, the β-chain gene locus contains two clusters each consisting of D and J segments: rearrangement first takes place in one of these and, if unsuccessful, the cell can attempt a rearrangement in the other cluster and then, if still unproductive, on the other chromosome. This means that many β-chain gene rearrangements are productive, and transcription follows to produce a β-chain expressed on the cell surface with a pTα-chain (equivalent to the surrogate light chain) and low amounts of CD3. As with B cells, this event triggers cell proliferation to produce many progeny, all expressing the same β-chain, and also blocks further β-chain gene rearrangement. At this stage, cells become double-positive (CD4+,CD8+) in preparation for selection, and express CD1 and CD38, and the transferrin receptor (CD71) which is needed for proliferation.

At the end of the proliferative stage, α-chain gene rearrangement begins involving V and J segments. Because there are so many J segments, each cell can attempt multiple rearrangements until one is successful. In some instances, productive rearrangements are seen on both chromosomes and the T cells express both combinations on the cell surface. RAG activity persists in the cell after completion of these rearrangements: it can promote further rearrangements in the α-chain gene while the cells are proceeding through positive selection thus affording more opportunities for selection and rescue from apoptosis. The overall result of this process is that there are many cells expressing the same β-chain but different α-chains thereby increasing the probability of cells expressing a particular β-chain being selected if useful to the host. Cells expressing the TCRs and CD3 at low density, accompanied by CD4+ and CD8+, enter positive selection (Fig. 6.9).

As with B cells, thymocytes die by apoptosis if they fail to make productive rearrangements in either their α- or β-chain genes.

Stem Cell
Precursor for T cells, NK cells and thymic dendritic cells
CD34+, CD44+, CD7+, CD25+(?)
↓
Double Negative Cell (CD4-CD8-)
β-gene rearrangements leading to expression
of pre-receptors **β-ptαlow, CD3low**
Further β-gene rearrangements blocked
CD34-, CD25-, CD71+, CD2+, 5+ and 7+
↓
PROLIFERATION
Double Positive Cell(CD4+CD8+)
α-gene rearrangement leads to many cells with
common β-chains paired with different α-chains
to give improved diversity for positive selection
expression of **TCRαβlow/CD3 low**
CD1+, CD38+, CD71-CD2+, 5+ & 7+
↓
POSITIVE SELECTION
(thymic epithelium)
↙   ↘

Cells which bind self MHC   Majority of cells do
(may involve more α-gene   not bind to MHC and
rearrangements) are rescued   undergo apopotosis
from cell death
CD1-, CD38-, CD71- **TCRαβhigh, CD3high**
CD2+, 5+, 7+, CD4+ OR CD8+
↓
NEGATIVE SELECTION
(thymic medulla by
macrophages/dendritic cells

↙   ↘

Cells which bind MHC-self peptide   Cells with **low affinity** for
with **medium/high affinity** undergo   MHC-self peptide move
apoptosis- removes potentially   to periphery as **helper(CD4+)**
autoreactive cells   and **cytotoxic** (CD8+) cells
                                          and recognize **MHCII-**
                                          foreign peptide
                                          CD2+, 5+, 7+, TCDαβ, CD3+
                                          CD4+ (TH) or CD8+ (TC)

Figure 6.9 – T cell maturation steps in the thymus. Only some major markers are shown.

Positive selection

Within the thymic cortex, the putative T cells come into contact with thymic epithelial cells expressing both MHC class I and II. The cells survive if they have undergone gene rearrangements to produce a TCR which successfully binds to either MHC I or II: the majority of cells that possess TCRs with no affinity for either MHC will undergo apoptosis. It is thought that during this process CD4 or CD8 aids the binding of TCR to MHC and this probably determines whether the cell becomes a CD4+ or a CD8+, i.e. they exhibit MHC I restriction or MHC II restriction. The cells cease expression of CD1 and CD38, and express TCR + CD3 and either CD4 or CD8 at high density in preparation for negative selection in the thymic medulla.

Negative selection

The positively selected cells migrate to the thymic medulla where there is a predominance of macrophages and interdigitating dendritic cells which express MHC class I and II and the full spectrum of self-peptides. These are, of course, the self-peptides that would be expressed on antigen-presenting cells in the periphery. The developing T cells interact with these antigen-presenting cells in the medulla: those cells (autoreactive CD4+ and CD8+) that bind with medium-to-high affinity to MHC-self peptide, i.e. exceed the activation threshold of the cell, undergo apoptosis and are removed. The cells that survive this selection emigrate from the thymus as mature helper and cytotoxic T cells, which will only be activated when they recognize self-MHC with bound foreign peptide, i.e. replacement of the self peptide with foreign peptide increases the affinity of binding above the activation threshold of the cell.

Mechanisms operative in positive and negative selection

Much effort has gone into the elucidation of the mechanisms by which T cells are selected by positive selection on thymic epithelial cells and by negative selection on haematopoietic cells (principally macrophages and dendritic cells). The major question relates to how interaction of TCR with the same ligand – MHC-self peptide – in positive selection leads to cell survival, while it leads to apoptosis in negative selection.

One possibility is that positive selection is, to a great extent, peptide independent. This suggests that although MHC expression requires peptide binding, the only required interactions are between TCR and MHC with interactions between TCR and the peptide being minimal. This process would positively select all cells that had any TCR-associated affinity for MHC and they would be rescued from cell death. As indicated earlier, CD4 and CD8 may enhance this binding. This population of cells would obviously include many capable of binding the particular MHC when bound to self-peptide and so presentation of these complexes by macrophages or dendritic cells during negative selection would promote their elimination, thus removing autoreactive cells.

Several years ago Marrack and Kappler suggested what has become known as 'the altered ligand hypothesis', which is based on the preceding suggestion. They proposed that there are ubiquitous peptides, unique to the thymus, which when bound to MHC I or II promote positive selection. In such situations it would seem the peptide is irrelevant and simply fulfills a structural requirement to stabilize the MHC and allow TCR interactions. The T cells, when encountering macrophages or dendritic cells, see the same MHC molecules but with a different set of self-peptides – the ones normally expressed in the periphery. TCR binding would then involve interactions with both MHC and peptide, with some T cells binding the complex with medium-to-high affinity, so becoming activated. These cells would be autoreactive in the periphery and would therefore undergo apoptosis.

The T cells remaining after these two events will be those that bind MHC self-peptide with low affinity, i.e. below the activation threshold of the cell, so they would not be activated by MHC self-peptide in the periphery. However, substitution of the self-peptide by foreign peptide could modify the ligand, thus enabling these cells to bind the complex with increased affinity and to undergo activation.

This model was in agreement with many of the then-current observations, but some objections have been raised more recently. These include the observation that, in rare cases, haematopoietic cells mediate positive selection and that certain peptides, when added to foetal thymic organ cultures, are found to bind to MHC on both epithelial and dendritic cells. In addition, analyses of peptides from thymic and other tissues have not shown any major differences in expression. However, recent work by Van Santen and colleagues suggests that empty MHC I molecules can mediate positive selection: this finding, together with a recent demonstration by Marrack and Kappler's laboratory that a single peptide can positively select a nearly complete T cell repertoire, supports their original ideas.

An alternative view is promulgated in what is now known as the 'signalling hypothesis', based on the phenotypes of the cells at various stages of development. Double-positive thymocytes that undergo positive selection only express low levels of TCR and CD3: in contrast, single-positive cells undergoing negative selection express high levels of both. It is known that to induce activation, at least 100 TCRs need to interact with an equal number of MHC–peptide complexes (all identical) at the point of cell contact. It is therefore perhaps reasonable to conclude that the density of TCRs and CD3s is too low to fulfill this requirement during positive selection, so cells are rescued from cell death by a much lower density which cannot result in activation even if the TCR is specific for MHC self-peptide. This would result in all cells exhibiting any binding to survive this process. However, during negative selection, single-positive cells will fulfill this requirement, and cells with TCRs binding MHC self-peptide with medium-to-high affinity will exceed the activation threshold. It is assumed activation signals must induce programmed cell death (i.e. apoptosis) leading to disposal of autoreactive cells.

A variation on this view is that positive or negative selection is determined partly by the amount of peptide available for presentation: experiments have shown that small amounts of peptides in thymic organ cultures lead to positive selection, whereas higher concentrations favour negative selection. Since there are many interactions between T cells and MHC-presenting cells, it would be expected that the density and affinity for the TCR, the density of the MHC-peptide, the presence of CD4 and/or CD8 and other cell adhesion molecules would all contribute to the final outcome.

Role of CDRs in binding MHC and peptide

TCR chains have to exhibit specificity for two components in the ligand – MHC and peptide. Once selected in the thymus, T cell specificity for MHC has to remain constant throughout the life of the T cell, and all T cells which bind to a particular MHC molecule must have a very similar specificity for the MHC part of the complex. However, each MHC allelic product binds many different peptides (estimated at 2000 in one study), so each individual T cell has to exhibit variations in specificity to accomodate this variability.

Until recently it was thought that each individual T cell selected in the thymus deals with this 'dual' specificity requirement by using CDR1 and CDR2 for binding to the MHC and CDR3 for binding to the peptide. However, recent crystallographic studies of the orientation of TCR in contact with HLA-A2-viral peptide suggest that CDR1 and CDR3 of both TCR chains bind peptide. Additionally, whereas all three CDRs of TCRα bind MHC, only CDR3 of TCRβ performs this task. It has therefore been suggested that the major bias of TCR is to bind to MHC, and this would explain the finding that a single peptide could select a nearly normal TCR repertoire and peptides, presumably increasing the affinity of binding and resulting in either partial or total activation in the periphery.

Extra-thymic tolerance induction

The thymus is the major site of development of T cells, and tolerance is induced through negative selection to self-peptides expressed by antigen-presenting cells and also many other major soluble self-components (blood proteins, etc.) delivered to the thymus. Nevertheless, there are other self-components, including those confined to fixed-cell populations in extra-thymic tissues, to which thymus-matured T cells have not been rendered tolerant. The question is how such tolerance arises when it is assumed that some positively selected T cells escape negative selection and which are therefore potentially auto-aggressive cells. Several theories have been proposed to explain this conundrum:

- the auto-antigen may not prime T_H cells as it is not expressed by the interdigitating dendritic cells which are the classical antigen-presenting cells that prime these T cells;

- the concentration of auto-antigen-derived peptides may be too low to stimulate T cells: note the requirement (discussed above) that at least 100 TCRs need to be occupied by MHC–peptide complexes for activation to occur;

- cells may not express MHC II thus blocking, in many cases, activation of both CD4+ and CD8+ cells;

- alternatively, cells may not deliver a costimulatory signal since they do not express B7 surface molecules. Thus the T cell response would fail resulting in anergy; and

- suppressor T cells may prevent either activation of CD4+ cells or inhibit cytokine function.

Extrathymic maturation of T cells

The existence of intestinal intraepithelial lymphocytes (IEL) in the gut has been known for a long time. However, in recent years it has been established that some of these T cells are not thymus-dependent but undergo maturation in the gut. These cells represent a major population of T cells, in fact the total numbers are about the same as all peripheral T cells in the spleen and lymph nodes, and show considerable heterogeneity in phenotype.

About half of the IEL are classical thymus-derived cells, predominantly CD8+, whereas the other half consist mostly of cells expressing CD8 α-chain homodimers, while some are double-negative cells expressing either αβ or γδ TCRs. (In contrast, thymus-derived cells express the conventional CD8 molecule consisting of an α and β chain.) It is thought that these double-negative cells, which probably arise from thymus-derived stem cells, undergo development in the gut. The contribution of T cell progenitors from the thymus was demonstrated when ectopic grafts of foetal thymus into the neonatally thymectomized or nude mouse dramatically increased the numbers of these 'thymus-independent' cells. If the gut is a totally thymus-independent environment for T cell maturation, then IEL should be detected in the nude mouse but they are generally not observed except in the older animal.

Although the mechanisms are still far from clear, studies in the transgenic mouse suggest that some form of positive and negative selection operates in the gut. It is perhaps important to observe that many of the thymus-independent IEL are potentially autoreactive. Furthermore, most IELs – both thymus- and gut-derived – are in an activated state and produce higher levels of cytokines than splenic T cells, and are associated with much cell death. This might suggest that IEL are selected by persistent antigens in the gut and it is perhaps a reasonable assumption that these cells are specific for the huge repertoire of antigens found in this tissue.

It has not yet been determined if IEL are involved in isotype switching of B cells to IgA production, although such a possibility is strongly suggested by the demonstration that CD8+ (as well as CD4+) IEL release IL-5 which can augment IgA production. In the near future, IEL will be better characterized and their functions delineated, and it may be that further extrathymic sites of T cell differentiation will be discovered.

CONCLUSIONS

Our understanding of B and T cell development is becoming clearer, although the early events underlying selection of T and B lineage by progenitor cells are still extremely poor. Most of the information will inevitably come from the transgenic or knock-out mouse and not from man, although quite a lot of early information was derived from the immunodeficient patient. The more recent information implying extrathymic maturation is interesting but very incomplete since the nature of the antigens which may promote extrathymic maturation is still not known: how this could affect clinical outcomes (in, for instance, transplantation) is currently speculative.

Based on our present understanding of T cell development, it would seem that immature cells from any individual could be used to reconstitute a patient since these cells would develop in the thymus and only those cells which developed suitable receptors for the recipient MHC would survive. However, it is known that even with matching for the MHC, especially MHC class II which controls T helper cells, there is a 10–20% failure to engraft – the reasons for this are not known. In cases where the recipient is lethally irradiated to kill host lymphoid cells or for a patient with SCID (severe combined immunodeficiency), it is essential for the graft to share some MHC alleles with the recipient. This is because the T cells that have adapted to host MHC recognition need professional antigen-presenting cells for activation, and their source is from the graft not the recipient. These APCs must therefore express some of the recipient MHC allelic products. There is also a danger of graft-versus-host reactions by mature T cells in the graft which have post-thymically migrated back to the bone marrow in the donor. These cells would recognize the recipient tissues as foreign and attempt to destroy it, and they have to be purged from the marrow before engraftment.

Methods for isolation of stem cells from bone marrow or blood are being developed, and this population, rather than whole bone marrow, may have a much better chance of success. Additionally, administration of some cytokines, such as granulocyte-macrophage colony stimulating factor, dramatically increases stem cell engraftment. It must be noted, however, that stem cells express donor-type MHC on their surfaces so any immunocompetence by the recipient may induce a transplantation reaction against the graft.

ADDITIONAL READING FOR MORE DETAILED INFORMATION

B cell development

An excellent, well-written, up-to-date account on every aspect of B cell development:
Janeway CA, Travers P. Immunobiology: the immune system in health and disease. Edinburgh: Churchill-Livingstone, 1996, pp. 5.1–29

A paper explaining the current understanding of how these different chains regulate B cell development:
Melchers F, Haasner D, Grawunder U et al. The role of IgH and L chains and of surrogate light chains in the development of cells of the B cell lineage. *Annual Reviews of Immunology* 1994; **12**: 209–225

A paper discussing in full the current idea of B cells changing their receptor affinity to survive antigen selection in the periphery:
Wagner SD, Neuberger MS. Somatic hypermutation of immunoglobulin genes. *Annual Reviews of Immunology* 1996; **14**: 441–457

T cell development

A chapter describing in detail, with excellent illustrations, every up-to-date aspect of T cell development:
Janeway CA, Travers P. Immunobiology: the immune system in health and disease. Edinburgh: Churchill-Livingstone, 1996, pp. 6.1–33

A current review of our knowledge on what occurs in the thymic cortex during the early stages of thymic education and which results in selection of MHC-recognizing T cells from the vast pool of T cells that have just undergone TCR DNA rearrangement:
Guidos CJ. Positive selection of CD4+ and CD8+ T cells. *Current Opinions in Immunology* 1996; **8**: 225–232

An easy-read paper about some of the important discoveries about the nature of the T cell receptor. It provides essential background to the present review:
Marrack P, Kappler J. The T cell receptor. *Science* 1987; **238**: 1073–1079

An important discussion on the nature of the peptide ligand which participates in the positive selection of thymocytes:
Hogquist KA, Jameson SC, Bevan MJ. The ligand for positive selection of T lymphocytes in the thymus. *Current Opinions in Immunology* 1994; **6**: 273–278

A timely reminder that not all T cells develop in the thymus. This review provides an update on current experimental evidence supporting the idea that the gut plays an important role especially in the development of γ-δ T cells:
Rocha B, Guy-Grand D, Vassalli P. Extrathymic T cell differentiation. *Current Opinions in Immunology* 1995; **7**: 235–242

A short review describing the results of a paper in the same issue of Nature *that sheds new light on the nature of the interaction between T cell receptors, MHC molecules and the peptide which is relevant to the discussion on T cell ontogeny:*
Parham P. Pictures of MHC restriction. *Nature* 1996; **384**: 109–103

7

PRODUCTION OF RECOMBINANT ERYTHROPOIETIN: A BRIEF HISTORY

C. D. R. Dunn and S. A. Marriott

SUMMARY

This chapter provides a starting point for those wishing to learn the basics of recombinant DNA technology as it has been applied to the production of erythropoietin (Epo) — 'the haematologists' hormone!' The paper is divided into four parts, the first of which outlines the generic conditions for any material to be produced using recombinant DNA technology. The second part provides an overview of the history of the development of Epo from a difficult-to-measure laboratory curiosity to the stage when production by recombinant technology was feasible. The third part collates these preceding parts to highlight how Epo was produced synthetically. The short, concluding, fourth part outlines the current and potential clinical applications of recombinant human Epo.

ESSENTIAL REQUIREMENTS FOR PRODUCTION OF A RECOMBINANT PROTEIN

Isolation of the gene

At least, in theoretical terms, production of a recombinant protein starts with isolation of the pure material (the protein itself), identification of its mRNA and, through the use of the enzyme reverse transcriptase, production of the complementary DNA (cDNA). The cDNA is then converted to double-stranded DNA, inserted in a vector and transferred into an appropriate host. After proliferation of the host cells, the resulting clones are screened to identify those containing the required gene.

In practice, this method is not always possible through lack of pure material and/or mRNA and, indeed, may not always be the preferred technique. In such circumstances, an alternative approach – 'shot-gun cloning' from a genomic library – may be employed. This involves the production of fragments of the entire genome using either restriction enzymes (partial digestion of genomic DNA which yields DNA fragments of varying lengths) or random shearing which produces fragments of around 20kb. The fragments are then inserted, one fragment per vector, in an appropriate cloning vehicle or vector, amplified in a suitable host cell and the desired gene traced to individual clones using a screening procedure such as hybridization with a radiolabelled nucleic acid probe.

Because 'shot-gun cloning' generates random-sized fragments of DNA, overlapping regions of the genome will be produced thus ensuring that every gene will be present in at least one fragment. Furthermore, because the fragments are relatively large, it is probable that large genes (or related, clustered, genes) will be present in their entirety. Alternatively, if the relevant gene can be localized to a particular fragment, it can be separated by a variety of analytical techniques (HPLC, density gradient centrifugation, agarose gel electrophoresis), and cloned as a smaller group of fragments.

Incorporation of the gene in a vector

Once the gene has been isolated it can be amplified/multiplied by molecular cloning, the first step of which is insertion of the gene (in the correct orientation) into an appropriate vector – a bacteriophage (phage), cosmid or plasmid. All of these 'replicons' can replicate independently. Phage vectors are derived from the *Escherichia coli* lambda phage in which each viral particle consists of a linear duplex of DNA packaged in a protein head, with a tubular protein tail and tail fibre. Each head can package 50kb DNA and at the 5' ends of each fragment are single-stranded sections of DNA (12bp) which are complimentary to each other – the so-called cos ends.

Cosmids can be thought of as a cross between plasmids and phage vectors: they are basically plasmids that contain the cos ends from the lambda phage and can therefore carry larger fragments of DNA. Although the choice of vector depends to some extent on the size of the gene to be inserted – cosmids can carrying genes ≤ 50kb – plasmid cloning in bacteria is by far the most commonly used process and is described here in more detail.

To be efficient, plasmid vectors need to be small, contain markers that allow them to be subsequently identified in cell clones, and to have unique recognition sites for restriction enzymes in a region not essential for plasmid replication.

The original plasmid vector, pBR322, contains genes coding for both tetracycline and ampicillin resistance, and was constructed such that cleavage sites for certain restriction enzymes occur only once. There are many vectors available for the cloning of DNA fragments and lots are based on pBR322 but which overcome its two main disadvantages: the few unique restriction sites, and the lengthy selection process. The limitation of restriction sites was overcome by the creation of a short sequence of DNA called the 'multiple cloning site' (MCS) located downstream of the regulatable segment of the *lacZ'* gene. This gene is regulated by the *lacI* gene situated downstream of the MCS. Overcoming the lengthy selection process involved the production of an active β-galactosidase which can hydrolyse the substrate 5-bromo-4-chloroindoyly-β-galactoside (X-gal) to a blue product. If the vector contained an insert then the X-gal would not be hydrolysed and the resulting product would be white.

Three procedures are commonly used to insert the relevant gene into the plasmid:

- homopolymer tailing occurs during the production of cDNA from mRNA using an oligo (dT) primer. This tail can be digested to give sticky ends and can be used in directional cloning. During the formation of the PCR product the enzyme usually incorporates an extra adenine base which can be used for cloning the PCR product on the 3' end into vectors which have been constructed to contain a 5' T overhang to complement the 3' A overhang;

- 'Linker cloning' or 'adapter cloning' involves the addition of a synthetic double-stranded oligonucleotide fragment to the ends of the cDNA whose base sequence specifies a particular restriction enzyme site. Adapters are constructed from two oligonucleotides of different lengths and can contain more than one restriction site. The process involves the preparation, using polymerase and exonuclease enzymes, of a cDNA fragment with blunt ends; separate incubations, in the presence of DNA ligase, of open plasmid and cDNA with a large excess of the double-stranded linker/adapter molecule; cleavage of both cDNA and plasmid using the appropriate restriction enzyme; and mixing of the cDNA and plasmid whereupon pairing occurs of cohesive complementary ends; and

- blunt-ended ligation can be considered as a modification of 'linker cloning' in which blunt ended fragments of the DNA are produced directly using an appropriate restriction enzyme. Such fragments can be ligated directly to the plasmid in a rather inefficient process, or ligated using the steps identified above.

During the gene insertion process, steps have to be taken to ensure that re-circularization of the plasmid only occurs after the gene has been incorporated. This can be accomplished using a DNA ligase which will only catalyse bond formation if one end of the DNA contains a 5'-phosphate and the other a 3'-OH moiety.

Transfer of the vector to the host

From the point of view of bulk production of the gene product, appropriate hosts for the vector include bacteria, yeast, continuous cell lines of mammalian origin and plants.

Of the various bacteria employed in recombinant DNA work, the K12 strain of *E. coli* and its derivatives are the most popular largely because their genetics are well understood. Transfer of the vector into the bacterial cells is accomplished by incubation at high temperature (42°C) and with calcium chloride which render the bacterial membrane permeable to the plasmid. This process is known as transformation.

Despite the convenience of *E. coli*, it is unable to undertake some types of processing (e.g. glycosylation) required of eukaryotic proteins and, for scale-up to commercial production, other species such as *Bacillus* are widely used, often with other types of vectors. Of such vectors, transposons – genetic elements which can be integrated into the host chromosome – can produce genes that are far more stably inherited than those transferred using a plasmid.

Bacteria carrying the vector can be identified in several ways:

- if the vector is tagged with a gene encoding antibiotic resistance, the bacteria can be grown in media containing the appropriate antibiotic;

- radioactive mRNA hybridization involves extraction of a few cells from each bacterial clone and, using ^{125}I-labelled mRNA, identifying those with the relevant DNA. The original clone can then be removed from the master plate and grown in a separate culture; and

- expression cloning involves cloning the DNA insert into 3'-end of the *E. coli lacZ* gene. This generates a reasonably stable fusion protein that can be detected with an appropriate antibody.

Yeasts represent the simplest eukaryotic system available for recombinant DNA work. Many species contain small, naturally occurring plasmids which will also propagate in *E. coli,* thus allowing the bacteria to be used in preliminary investigations. An important development was the construction of yeast artificial chromosomes (YACs) for cloning fragments of $0.1–1.0 \times 10^6$ bp.

In general, yeasts seem less able than bacteria to recognize foreign promoters and regulatory sequences such that expression of foreign proteins is not usually as efficient. Furthermore, as is typical of eukaryotes in general, gene expression in yeast is modulated by regulatory elements which may be many thousands of base pairs from the gene of interest. Yeasts do not usually excise introns from higher eukaryote DNA and thus are not that superior to bacteria in cloning genes from genomic libraries.

In theory, continuous cell lines of mammalian origin represent an effective expression system for human genes: in practice, they can be inefficient from an economical viewpoint because of their slower proliferation rate compared with bacteria and yeast. Mammalian cells can take up foreign DNA simply through adsorption – a process known as transfection – although this is not usually very efficient. Alternatively, the DNA can be introduced by microinjection or by inducing the cultured cells to fuse with DNA-containing vesicles such as liposomes or bacterial protoplasts. Transposons or plasmids encoding neomycin resistance can be used as vectors, as can tumour viruses (e.g. SV40) and various retroviruses. Of the latter, the mouse mammary tumour virus contains a promoter that can be turned on and off using glucocorticoids. Thus, for example, the culture can become established prior to 'switching on' production of the desired product.

Foreign genes can also be transferred to plant cells. Wounds on intact plants can be inoculated with the Ti plasmid carried by the tumour-forming bacterium *Agrobacterium tumefaciens*. The resulting tumours, like their mammalian counterparts, are relatively easy to culture with the recombinant cells containing Ti DNA randomly inserted in the host nuclear genome. However, for many of the more sophisticated studies, tumour formation is not particularly helpful so the Ti plasmid is often rendered non-oncogenic by deletion of the oncogenes.

Plant expression systems offer the advantages of economy and high yield. However, they cannot be induced to secrete large polypeptide and protein molecules.

Transgenic animals possibly represent the ultimate in gene expression systems. With these systems, microinjection techniques are used to integrate the foreign gene in the DNA of newly fertilized eggs so that it will be expressed in the adult animal. Tissue-specific gene expression is not yet sufficiently well understood for the technique to be completely reliable, but impressive results have been obtained in some instances, such as in the transgenic mouse which overproduces mouse or human growth hormone; expression of chicken transferrin in mouse; and, most dramatically, sheep which secretes human factor VIII into its milk.

Ultimately, the goal might be to transfer the isolated and properly controlled gene directly into the patient requiring therapy with the gene product. Although some have argued that goal is being approached rapidly, it remains on the horizon in so far as the Epo gene is concerned. Rather, the generation of small molecule agonists for the Epo receptor might be a more attractive medium-term goal (see below).

Expression of the gene *in vitro*

Production of the required product is often rather more complex than simply getting the gene in an appropriate host and letting it get on with the job! For example:

- the gene must be transcribed using a promoter that allows RNA polymerase to bind to DNA. This process is usually accomplished by inserting the gene into a vector 'downstream' from a bacterial promoter such as the ptac12 plasmid promoter. This promoter is also susceptible to induction (by adding lactose or IPTG) and repression thus allowing gene transcription to be controlled;

- in eukaryotes, an important step in gene transcription is the excision of introns – non-coding sections of DNA in the middle of genes. However, bacteria lack the ability to excise such material. This difficulty can be overcome by modifing the genomic DNA to exclude the introns prior to insertion (i.e. cDNA), or by employing a suitable eukaryotic expression system;

- translation of the mRNA coding for the required gene product requires the presence of a ribosomal binding site upstream from the initiation codon. Thus, the gene for this site must also be inserted in the vector;

- because eukaryotic genes do not always have easily identifiable transcription termination signals, when such a gene is expressed the appropriate termination codons must be added at the 3'-end; and

- a mechanism must be available to perform any post-translational modifications to which the required product is normally exposed. If not glycosylated (a process which bacteria cannot perform), many proteins are rapidly cleared from the circulation and thereby are relatively inactive. Other proteins such as insulin are only active after they are cleaved from the precursor gene product.

Extraction of the desired protein

Extracting the desired product from host cells can also present difficulties. If produced in bacteria such as *E. coli*, which does not secrete materials, the cells must be lysed by shearing, sonication or chemical treatment. While these procedures are effective, they also release endotoxins that have to be removed separately. Other bacteria, e.g. *Bacillus subtilis*, secrete gene products into the culture media and attempts are being made to utilize these secretion signals in the production of recombinant proteins. Once in the culture media, the products can be purified by conventional biochemical techniques such as affinity chromatography.

Scale-up to commercial production

The scaling-up of laboratory procedures to the level required of commercial production generally represents a formidable undertaking. It usually involves:

- production of the appropriately sized equipment;

- further refinements in the host organism to optimize production of the required product. The characteristics of an optimum industrial microorganism might include:

  - the ability to express eukaryotic genes;
  - a high copy number plasmid;
  - the capability of post-translational modifications (e.g. glycosylation);
  - the ability to secrete proteins in the surrounding media;
  - an inexpensive fermentation substrate;
  - a low order of pathogenicity;
  - weak antigenicity; and
  - strain stability meaning the organisms are relatively robust to minor variations in steady-state conditions;

- selection of the most appropriate substrate that, in many processes, is the largest cost factor;

- optimum design of the fermenter on which most commercial procedures to generate recombinant DNA products are based; and

- adaptation of the product recovery process.

The overall success of the process depends on three factors – optimization of production, economy and safety.

FROM LABORATORY CURIOSITY TO RECOMBINANT PRODUCT

Acceptance of the humoral regulation of erythropoiesis

The history of the recognition of Epo as an important regulator of erythropoiesis, and whose production was determined by some function of the oxygen concentration in inspired air, is often traced to the important studies reported by Carnot and Deflandre in 1906. In fact, it is possible to trace the concept of oxygen-mediated erythropoiesis before their seminal investigations.

By 1845 it was known that oxygen was an essential component of air, and that it was taken up by blood in the lungs. Hoppe-Seyler, in 1862, showed that oxygen was reversibly bound to haemoglobin, and this led to a general acceptance that red blood cells (RBCs) were of vital importance in oxygen transport.

In 1863, Jourdanet and Bert noted that many of their Mexican patients who moved from sea level to high altitude developed the symptoms of anaemia – weakness, shortness of breath and lightheadness – even though RBC counts were in the normal range or even increased in number. They also noted that the blood of patients who had adapted to altitude was extremely dark and flowed slowly over the operating table. However, no connection was made between the thickness of the patients' blood and the adaptation to the low oxygen pressure at high altitude.

Viault, in 1890, did make that connection when he observed an increase in his own RBC count when he travelled by train from Lima, Peru, to the tin mines of Morochocha at an altitude of 4400m above sea level. His RBC count increased from 5×10^6 to 7×10^6 mm^{-3} after 2 weeks, and to 8×10^6 mm^{-3} after 3 weeks' residence at Morochocha. Meischer, in Switzerland, extended these observations and suggested that hypoxia directly stimulated the bone marrow to produce more blood cells.

And then, in 1906, Carnot and Deflandre proposed an alternative hypothesis. Noting that serum from moderately anaemic rabbits produced an increased RBC count when infused into normal animals, they proposed that hypoxia indirectly stimulated RBC production through a circulating 'haemopoietin' produced in response to reduced oxygen tension sensed at a site outside of the bone marrow. However, numerous attempts by many different investigators generally failed to confirm Carnot and Deflandre's results and to detect this factor.

In 1950, Reissmann and colleagues using parabiotic rats showed that when one animal was exposed to hypoxia the partner also increased production of RBCs. Thus, some material was produced in one animal and was passed through the connected circulatory system into the partner, to stimulate RBC production. Stohlman, in 1954, came to the same conclusion from studies with a patient with a patent ductus arteriosus – where the foetal ductus arteriosus between pulmonary artery and aorta fails to close properly. The same degree of erythroid hyperplasia was apparent in both normal and cyanotic areas of the body suggesting a systemic effect (mediated by haemopoietin) to only local hypoxia.

But the first direct evidence of an erythroid stimulating factor in the plasma of anaemic or hypoxic animals was reported in 1953 by Erslev. He transfused large volumes (50ml per day for 4 or 5 days) of plasma from rabbits with blood loss anaemia to normal animals and showed increases in peripheral blood reticulocytes and marrow normoblasts, and a somewhat slower increase in haematocrit and RBC count. The active erythroid stimulating factor was renamed 'erythropoietin' as haematopoietic stimulation seemed specific for erythropoiesis.

Having produced evidence generally in support of the presence of Epo, the next questions that needed to be considered were: where was it produced and on what cells did it act?

Production of erythropoietin

Hypoxia is obviously the trigger for Epo production. Even in the mid–late 1950s it was known that Epo was present in plasma and urine (at least in anaemic states) and that its concentration was proportional to the degree of hypoxia (anaemia). Furthermore, many data from this type of study added support to the concept that Epo was not only a trigger for RBC production, but also was responsible for the overall regulation of RBC production in the normal physiological situation.

Theoretical considerations about the possible site for a hypoxia sensor indicated that some organs – e.g. heart, brain and liver – could be excluded because of compensatory systems involving the redistribution of blood to hypoxic areas. On the other hand, organs that became relatively hypoxic because of this redistribution, e.g. the subcutaneous tissue and the kidneys, might be good candidates. For a variety of reasons – extensive blood supply and relatively small oxygen requirements – the kidney appeared the less suitable of these two possibilities.

However, Jacobson et al in 1957 showed in a series of extirpation studies that the kidney was the major site of production of Epo. The anephric rat failed to respond to anaemia by producing RBCs, while the 'nephric' rat (its kidneys intact but the ureters ligated) responded normally. Thus, the erythroid regulatory role of the kidney was also shown to be distinct from its excretory functions. In the foetus, the liver seems to be the primary source of Epo, and this organ can produce very limited amounts (and with poor sensitivity to hypoxia) in the absence of kidneys in the adult. In addition, the carotid body has been shown to have the biochemical machinery to produce Epo, although its role in erythropoiesis remains uncertain (and is probably minimal).

Despite Jacobson et al's data, subsequent studies by several groups of investigators generally failed to either extract active Epo from the kidney or to produce the hormone in cell culture. Furthermore, this general failure applied to kidneys or cells from normal animals, as well as those from animals in which Epo production had been triggered by short periods of hypoxia or blood loss anaemia. These failings contribute to the reasons why – 40 years after Jacobson et al's studies – it is still not known with certainty which renal cells produce Epo (although it is probably tubular or peritubular cells), and whether Epo is secreted as the active molecule (most probably) or as an inactive precursor which has to undergo enzymatic conversion to an active form in the circulation. Nevertheless, there is compelling evidence that a hypoxia sensor, activation of which increases the synthesis of Epo, depends on an oxygen-sensitive NAD(P)H-oxidase within the haem protein cytochrome b_{558} of the cell membrane.

Depending on the partial pressure of oxygen on haemoglobin (pO_2), oxygen radicals are produced that are converted to H_2O_2, which acts as a second messenger. By 'scavenging' H_2O_2 either through glutathione peroxidase or catalase, guanylate cyclase is activated, leading to a change in the relative amounts of reduced:oxidized glutathione (2GSH:GSSG) or cGMP. This change, among others, activates potassium channels and cytosolic transcription factors that specifically bind to enhancing elements in the cell to initiate enhanced expression of the constitutively active Epo gene on chromosome 7.

This system does not depend on oxygen bound to haemoglobin as atmospheric oxygen will modulate the receptor directly. Furthermore, it can explain how nickel and cobalt increase Epo production: they replace ferrous iron in newly synthesized porphyrin rings of the cytochrome resulting in the substituted haem protein behaving like native deoxygenated iron haem by modifying the availability of oxygen and changing the ratio of 2GSH: GSSG in favour of increased Epo production. Potassium channels are thought to be important in getting newly synthesized Epo out of the cells. Interestingly, similar oxygen-sensing systems have been recognized in many cell types (including some within the CNS), and it is not clear why some cells actually liberate Epo and others have the machinery to do so but apparently do not!

It appears that human Epo is synthesized as a 193 amino acid polypeptide that undergoes a series of post-translational modifications. A 27 amino acid leader sequence is cleaved to give a 166 amino acid form, and the C-terminal arginine residue at 166 is removed possibly by an intracellular carboxypeptidase. Finally, the peptide undergoes glycosylation through N-linkage at asparagine residues 24, 38 and 83 and O-linkage at serine 126 to produce the complete Epo protein with a molecular weight of 30.4kDa.

Site of action of erythropoietin

Detailed discussion of the site of action of Epo is really beyond the scope of this review. However, it is worth noting that the rate of production of RBCs can increase by at least a factor of 10. Therefore, erythroid precursors must normally be turning over fairly slowly to have sufficient reserve to meet extra demands. However, examination of morphologically recognizable RBC precursors in marrow indicates that, even maximally stimulated, the increase in cell divisions would do no more than double, perhaps quadruple, the output of mature cells. Finally, the time delay (2–4 days) between application of a stimulus and a significant erythropoietic response (reticulocytosis and increased haematocrit) led to the suggestion that Epo acted on 'stem cells' which, in the 1960s, were operationally defined as erythropoietin-responsive cells.

Further elaboration of the characteristics of these cells awaited the development by Axelrad's group in Toronto in 1973 of the *in vitro* growth of erythroid colonies in much the same way that colonies of granulocytes and/or macrophages had been cultured since the mid-1960s. The outcome of numerous studies since 1973 suggest that while Epo has several sites of action on both erythroblastic and possibly megakaryoblastic cells within the haematopoietic stem cell compartment (and perhaps on mature cells), its principal site of action appears to be on the cells CFU-E, defined by their ability to produce small colonies of erythrocytic cells *in vitro*. As circulating titres of Epo increase, CFU-E respond quickly by proliferation and differentiation and, as Epo titres decline, the cells undergo apoptosis and the erythroid response is attenuated.

The mRNA encoding the Epo receptor is transcribed from the receptor gene in a process dependent on GATA-1 (a haematopoietic transcription factor) and other transcription factors. Translation of the mRNA results in a 62kDa peptide glycosylated to a 64kDa form in the endoplasmic reticulum. During transit through the Golgi body, the receptor is further glycosylated to a 66kDa form. The addition of more carbohydrate to the receptor results in it appearing on the cell surface in forms with molecular weights in the range 70–78kDa, and with a 105kDa form which may be required for receptor activation. Of the 70–78kDa forms, only the 78kDa type becomes phosphorylated on tyrosine residues, and that only occurs after binding to Epo – the receptor does not have a recognizable kinase domain, so it would appear that the 78kDa subunit interacts with a tyrosine protein kinase only after Epo has bound. This results in the receptor and some other proteins becoming phosphorylated, and one or more of these phosphorylated proteins may be responsible for activating nuclear events associated with the biological activity of Epo. Furthermore, activation of the receptor may be associated with the formation of receptor dimers.

The interaction between Epo and its receptors on target cells is fairly typical of hormone:target cell interactions. Following Epo binding, the receptor:Epo complex is endocytosed and destroyed. Considerable evidence suggests that Epo-dependent activation of tyrosine kinase and phosphoinositide 3 (IP_3)-kinase are important components of the intracellular pathway in an apparently similar way to several other haematopoietic growth factors and cytokines. Single amino acid substitutions in the receptor can result in inactivation.

Between 100 and 1,000 Epo receptors are expressed per RBC precursor but some erythroleukaemia cell lines may have 10,000 receptors per cell. The receptor affinity varies from 10pm to 1nm with evidence for two receptor subtypes with high and low affinity. Nevertheless, what controls their relative expression is unknown, and the importance of any differential functional significance is not yet fully appreciated. It is possible that receptor numbers and their affinities may vary with the maturation stage of the erythroid precursors. It is known, for example, that at the usually low physiological levels of Epo more hormone is bound to cells having the high- rather than the low-affinity receptors. The Epo receptor may contain both growth-promoting (viability/proliferation) and differentiation-promoting activities: polypeptides designated AIC2A and AIC2B are associated with Epo-dependent cell proliferation (by activation of genes like *c-myc*, *egr-1*, *c-fos*), with some additional data suggesting that the cytoplasmic part of the Epo receptor has a specific differentiation domain that controls the accumulation of β-globin.

PRODUCTION OF RECOMBINANT ERYTHROPOIETIN

Several significant factors delayed the production of Epo using recombinant DNA technology. Low endogenous levels in plasma (of the order of 0.1ng/ml) and the urine of normal subjects, and failure to extract Epo even from 'triggered' tissues, raised the possibility of the synthesis of an inactive precursor which required enzymatic action to produce active material. The importance of glycosylation in delaying excretion of Epo was recognized in the 1960s, and in some ways this diverted attention away from the purification of the hormone to a discussion of the relative merits of *in vivo* (detecting only glycosylated material) and *in vitro* (detecting both glycosylated and un-glycosylated material) assays. But probably the most important handicaps from a synthetic viewpoint were the absence of 'pure' Epo; the lack of a cell line that *in vitro* consistently produced the hormone (and from which mRNA might therefore be extracted); and a lack of understanding of the mode of induction of Epo synthesis and release. Was it, for example, produced constitutively, on demand, or released from a storage site?

Dedicated work by, first, Goldwasser and Kung, in 1971, with the plasma of anaemic sheep and, second, by Miyake and colleagues, in 1977, eventually led to the purification of Epo. Miyake *et al* started with a total volume of 2,550 litres of pooled urines, collected mostly from patients with aplastic anaemia, and estimated to contain 1–6U/ml Epo. They subjected this material to a seven-step procedure during which Epo was purified by a factor of 930 to give a 'pure' product of specific activity 10,400U/mg with a 25% yield. Two fractions of the same potency and molecular size, but differing slightly in electrophoretic mobility at pH9, were obtained although the significance of these fractions was (and remains) uncertain.

The magnitude of the problem of purifying Epo can be appreciated from some straightforward calculations. Assuming Miyake *et al*'s product was 'pure', a specific activity of 10,400U/mg means that the group's starting material contained around 0.5μg/ml Epo: if 'pure' Epo has a specific activity of 129,000U/mg (when produced in COS cells; see below), then the starting material contained around 40pg/ml Epo. Normal human plasma is generally considered to contain around 20mU/ml Epo: *c.*3 or 0.2pg/ml depending on whether the specific activity is 10,400 or 129,000U/mg respectively. (One unit of biological activity of Epo was originally defined as the erythropoietic effect of $5\mu M$ $CoCl_2$ in the *in vivo* fasted rat bioassay, but now corresponds to a unit in the International Reference Preparation held at the National Institute for Biological Standards and Control in London, UK.)

The three-dimensional structure (by X-ray crystallography) of Epo has not yet been determined, and the biological features of the molecule that confer its activity are still largely unknown. It has been proposed, based largely on comparisons with growth hormone and cytokines, that Epo consists of a four-membered α-helical bundle with interconnecting loops. All four helices (arranged in an 'up-up-down-down' folding pattern) are required for biological activity as are the disulphide bridges linking the N- and C-termini. Charged and neutral amino acids on each helix are exposed at the surface, while hydrophobic residues are located inside the structure. There is a high degree of homology of Epos from man, monkey, cat, dog, pig, sheep, mouse, and rat.

In 1985, Saito et al described the translation of mRNA from a renal tumour to a product with the biological properties of Epo, and two groups described the full synthesis of Epo using recombinant DNA technology. Lin et al (1985) subjected purified human urinary Epo to tryptic digestion, followed by isolation and microsequencing of the fragments. Despite some uncertainties, particularly about the first 23 amino-terminal positions, some definitive amino acid sequences were obtained. These allowed the construction of 20-mer (base) and 17-mer oligonucleotides containing all possible sequences that could code for the selected amino acid sequences: each set of oligonucleotide probes contained a pool of 128 sequences. Using these oligonucleotides, a human foetal liver genomic library in the bacteriophage vector Charon 4A was screened (using the 'shot gun' approach; see above) for the gene coding for Epo. Among the library of 1,500,000 clones screened, the 20-mer probe hybridized to 272 phage plaques and the 17-mer probe to around 4,000. However, only four plaques hybridized with both probes. Southern blot and DNA sequence analyses showed that three of these clones contained at least a portion of the Epo gene, while the fourth – λHE1 – contained the complete gene the protein-coding region of which was divided into four introns and five exons. Through a comparison with the amino acid sequence of human urinary Epo it was possible to identify the nucleotide sequence in the gene exons. In turn, this allowed comparison of the genomic sequence to that in the cDNA derived from mRNA isolated from (mammalian) CHO (Chinese hamster ovary) cells, which were ultimately used to produce recombinant Epo.

Biologically active recombinant human Epo was produced in CHO cells that had been stably transformed with an expression vector containing the genomic Epo gene insert driven by the SV40 late promoter. A 'representative' sample of media from 5-day cultures contained 18.2U/ml Epo when measured by radioimmunoassay, and 15.8±4.6 and 16.8±3.0U/ml when measured by *in vitro* and *in vivo* bioassays respectively. The fact that the material showed similar activity in both bioassays strongly suggested that it was fully glycosylated – an observation confirmed by the finding that treatment of the secreted product with endo-β-N-acetylglucosaminidase F reduced the apparent molecular weight from 34 to c.19kDa.

Concluding, Lin et al claimed that their study represented the first time that mixed oligonucleotide probes had been used for the isolation of genes from mammalian genomic libraries. The study thus demonstrated a new avenue for the isolation of genomic sequences for which only limited quantities of pure product were available and no mRNA or specific antibody. The 'two-site' approach – using two oligonucleotides – eliminated many false-positives thus resulting in a 'great saving' in time, effort and money. Lin et al also emphasized the importance of optimization of each of the steps in the cloning procedure.

Jacobs et al (1985) also started with Epo purified according to the general method of Miyake et al and similarly subjected it to trypsin digestion. The digest was processed on a reverse-phase HPLC, well-separated peaks evaporated to dryness and subjected to N-terminal sequence analysis. Oligonucleotides were prepared to two of these fragments and, as in Lin et al's process, used to isolate the Epo gene from a bacteriophage λ library of human genomic DNA. The Epo genomic clones were then used to show that human foetal liver was a potential source of mRNA for cDNA cloning: material corresponding to an mRNA of approximately 1,600 nucleotides was detected. The same oligonucleotide probes were also used to isolate cDNA clones from a bacteriophage λ cDNA library construct from foetal liver. The complete nucleotide and deduced amino acid sequence for the largest of these clones – λHEPOFL13 – contained 579 nucleotides in the 5' half of the cDNA and encoded a hydrophobic 27-amino acid leader peptide followed by the 166-amino acid mature Epo protein.

As in Lin et al's study, the gene was found to consist of five exons with parts of exons I and V coding for the 5' and 3' untranslated sequences respectively. The gene was cloned into p91023B vector (which contains the adenovirus major late promoter, a simian virus (SV40) poly(A) sequence, an SV40 enhancer, and origin of replication and the adenovirus virus-associated gene), and expressed in COS cells.

Both Lin et al and Jacobs et al did not find any evidence to support the concept that biologically inactive forms of Epo were produced (see above). No promoter sequences were found anywhere in the gene, and neither were any consensus poly(A) signal sequences located. Furthermore, a computer-aided homology search of both monkey and human Epo genes against GenBank and the entire Dayhoff protein bank failed to reveal significant homology with any published DNA or protein sequences including angiotensinogen, which has been suggested as a possible Epo precursor. The secreted product produced by both groups showed similar activity in both *in vivo* and *in vitro*, and had an identical amino acid sequence to the authentic product. It has an isoelectric point of 4.2–4.6: non-glycosylated Epo from *E. coli* has an apparent pI of 9.2.

Presumably for commercial reasons, there is relatively little published data about how the laboratory-based synthesis of Epo was scaled-up for the manufacture of the peptide in sufficient quantities for clinical use. However, Egrie (1990) (from Lin's group) noted that scale-up involved insertion of the cloned Epo gene adjacent to a viral promoter in an expression vector that also contained the gene for dihydrofolate reductase (DHFR). The viral promoter enhanced gene expression by increasing the production of mRNA transcripts, while the DHFR gene provided a selectable marker and a means for gene amplification: conversion of DHFR-deficient CHO cells to DHFR+ phenotype by expression of the gene allowed their selection by culturing in the presence of methotrexate. After gene amplification, a single cell was isolated by limiting-dilution cloning, expanded in culture, and aliquots of several million cells stored frozen in a master working cell bank. Epo production from this bank involves thawing and culturing the contents of a single vial, followed, at appropriate (but unspecified) times, by isolation and purification of Epo using sequential chromatography. The final purified bulk product is formulated in 0.25% human serum albumin to prevent adsorption of Epo to surfaces from the relatively dilute solutions that make up the final dose forms. Each lot of the product is subjected to extensive specification testing to ensure identity, integrity, purity, sterility, biological activity and potency.

The product described by Lin et al is the basis for erythropoietin α (Eprex, with 31% carbohydrate) marketed by Amgen worldwide and by Cilag in the UK. The product produced by Jacobs et al is the basis for erythropoietin β (Recormon,

24% carbohydrate) marketed by Genetics Institute worldwide and by Boehringer Mannheim (now part of the Roche group) in the UK. Although they differ in carbohydrate content, they are deemed to be clinically indistinguishable and one or other or both preparations are now available in over 70 countries worldwide.

CLINICAL USES OF ERYTHROPOIETIN

Using crude preparations, studies by Van Dyke and colleagues in the 1960s provided tantalizing concepts of the clinical potential of pure Epo in the management of patients with chronic renal disease – a complaint in which treatment with Epo can be seen as a 'haematology hormone replacement therapy' – HHRT!

Given that the kidney is the primary site of Epo production and that renal disease is associated with a hypoproliferative anaemia, the anaemia of end-stage renal disease was the obvious first clinical target for recombinant human Epo. Two groups – Winearls et al (1986) in the UK and Eschbach et al (1987) in the USA – gained the plaudits for being the first to report that the recombinant human hormone could correct the anaemia of end-stage renal disease. In these first studies, Epo was given by thrice-weekly, bolus intravenous injections over the dose range of 3–500U/kg. Increases in reticulocyte counts, haematocrit, haemoglobin and iron utilization (and decreases in iron overload) all heralded correction of the anaemia and almost completely obviated transfusion dependence. Toxic reactions were few and far between although five of the total of 35 patients had some signs of hypertension and two had blood clots in their arteriovenous fistulas.

The results of these trials confirmed the expectation that Epo could increase the haematocrit in patients with end-stage renal disease and improve the patients' sense of well-being. Subsequent studies have generally shown that subcutaneous injections of Epo produce the same benefits as bolus intravenous dosing but with 20–30% lower total doses because the subcutaneous tissue acts as a depot from which hormone is released over protracted periods. Similarly, circulatory problems and hypertension can be minimized by ensuring only gradual increases in haematocrit to a value (in the range of 10–12g/dl for adult and 9.5–11g/dl for child) perhaps at the lower end of what is usually considered 'normal' for patients with functional kidneys. The usual recommendation is to start with thrice-weekly subcutaneous injections of 50U/kg and increase the dose in steps of 25U/kg at 4-week intervals to a maximum of 600U/kg/week in three doses. One or more of the doses should be omitted if the increase in haemoglobin concentration >2g/dl per month. For reasons that are not yet clear (functional iron or folate deficiency, or failure of dialysis to remove one or more erythroid toxins), a variable proportion of patients show 'resistance' to the effects of Epo and fail to respond with the expected correction of their anaemia.

While end-stage renal disease is the obvious clinical target for recombinant human Epo, it has also been shown to produce benefit in a variety of other refractory anaemias including those associated with chronic disease, AIDS and as a consequence of cytotoxic chemotherapy. Epo has also been used successfully to increase the yield of autologous blood (and thereby obviate the need for homologous transfusions) in predonation programmes for elective surgery. Suggestions that similar programmes have been used for autologous blood 'doping' by athletes are difficult to substantiate.

CONCLUSIONS

It was 44 years between Carnot and Deflandre's suggestion of the existence of Epo and experimental verification that such a factor existed. It then took about 20 years before the factor was purified; a further 9 years between purification and reports of gene cloning; and only 2 more years (in 1980–2) before recombinant Epo was being evaluated in man. And in the mid-1970s a better concept of what constituted the target cells for Epo was obtained.

Epo was not the first hormone or cytokine to be synthesized: that honour generally goes to insulin. Unlike insulin (which could be extracted from animals), no animal source of Epo was available and, in general, the only alternative therapy was repeated blood transfusions with the associated inconveniences and risks. Like insulin, there was a disorder – in Epo's case, the anaemia of end-stage renal disease – for which there was general expectation that the product would be clinically effective. That expectation was not misplaced, and, in the 10 years or so since the first detailed clinical trials, recombinant human Epo has gained an established place in the armamentarium of agents available to treat anaemias in which inappropriately low endogenous levels of the hormone contribute to the pathology. Like the colony stimulating factors (CSFs) used to minimize periods of neutropaenia after cytotoxic chemotherapy or bone marrow transplantation, Epo may not reduce mortality, but there seems little doubt that it improves patients' quality of life, minimizes hospital visits, and greatly reduces the inconvenience and risks (infection, iron overload) associated with repeated blood transfusions.

But science and medicine do not stand still. Pharmaceutical companies are already working on 'second generation' products that might be either small-molecule, orally active compounds which trigger (act as agonists at) Epo receptors, or which can activate Epo genes, presumably in organs such as the liver which might be functionally normal even in patients with end-stage renal disease. Additionally, injection of naked plasmids encoding Epo has been shown to stimulate erythrocyte production in the laboratory animal. No sooner have we got used to using Epo in the clinic, we can envisage its demise and replacement with compounds which achieve the same aims more simply and conveniently and, possibly, less expensively.

ACKNOWLEDGEMENTS

The work of Dr SA Marriott is generiously supported by a research grant from Amgen Ltd, Milton Rd Cambridge.

SELECTED READING FOR MORE DETAILED INFORMATION

Possibly the most important of two or three studies in the mid-1970s claiming the purification of human urinary Epo. Worth reviewing if only to gain an appreciation of the perseverance of the investigators:
Miyake T, Kung CKH, Goldwasser E. Purification of human erythropoietin. *Journal of Biological Chemistry* 1977; **252**: 5558–5564

Two good, overall reviews (the first by Lin's team: the second more from the perspective of Jacobs' group) of the synthesis of recombinant human Epo and of its properties:
Browne JK, Cohen AM, Egrie JC et al. Erythropoietin: gene cloning, protein structure, and biological properties. In Cold Spring Harbour Symposia on Quantitative Biology, vol. LI, 1986, pp. 693–702

Hirth P, Wieczorek L, Scigalla P. Molecular biology of erythropoietin. *Contr Nephrol* 1988; **66**: 38–53

These two references are the seminal reports of the synthesis of recombinant human Epo. The procedures used were essentially similar and, although Jacob et al's paper appeared first, the work must have been concurrent in both laboratories:
Jacobs K, Shoemaker C, Rudersdorf R et al. Isolation and characterisation of genomic and cDNA clones of human erythropoietin. *Nature* 1985; **313,** 806–810

Lin F-K, Suggs S, Lin C-H et al. Cloning and expression of the human erythropoietin gene. *Proceedings of the National Academy of Sciences, USA* 1985; **82**: 7580–7584

Perhaps the definitive report detailing the chemical structure of human urinary Epo to which recombinant material is compared:
Lai P-H, Everett R, Wang F-F et al. Structural characterization of human erythropoietin. *Journal of Biological Chemistry* 1986; **261**: 3116–3121

This multi-author book is almost a synopsis of 'everything you wanted to know about the synthesis and properties of recombinant human Epo but were afraid to ask!' It includes chapters with a historical perspective, it details the synthesis of Epo, and outlines many of the early important clinical trials. Essential reading to get the overall picture about Epo up to about 1990:
Erslev AJ, Adamson JW, Eschbach JW, Winearls C (eds). Erythropoietin: molecular, cellular, and clinical biology. The Johns Hopkins University Press, Baltimore and London, 1991

These two papers – the first from the UK, the second from the USA — represent the first reports of the clinical use of recombinant human Epo in patients with end-stage renal disease:
Winearls CG, Oliver DO, Pippard MJ et al. Effect of human erythropoietin derived from recombinant DNA on the anaemia of patients maintained by chronic haemodialysis. *Lancet* 1986; **II**: 1175–1178
Eschbach JW, Egrie JC, Downing MR et al. Correction of the anemia of end-stage renal disease with recombinant human erythropoietin. *New England Journal of Medicine* 1987; **316**: 73–78

These four books are representative of a plethora of texts on biotechnology: the second is particularly useful as it focuses as much on scale-up procedures, manufacturing and finance as it does on more laboratory-based biotechnology:
Brown TA. Gene cloning: An introduction, 2nd edn. London: Chapman & Hall, 1990

Moses V, Cape RE. Biotechnology: the science and the business. London: Harwood, 1991

Moses V, Moses S. Exploiting biotechnology. London: Harwood, 1995

Balasubramanian D, Bryce CFA, Dharmalingam K et al. Concepts in biotechnology. London: Sangam, 1996

This ring-bound book contains lots of up-to-date and useful information on haematology in an easy-to-assimilate, tutorial, note-taking style with plenty of informative figures. Well worth obtaining as a 'banker' text for haematology generally!:
Israels LG, Israels ED. Mechanisms in hematology. Winnipeg: University of Manitoba, 1996

One of the few papers discussing the scale-up of Epo production from laboratory to manufacture for clinical use:
Egrie J. The cloning and production of recombinant human erythropoietin. *Pharmacotherapy* 1990; **10**: 3S–8S

A good review of the relative benefits of different dose regimens and routes of administration:
Ashai NI, Paganini EP, Wilson JM. Intravenous versus subcutaneous dosing of epoetin: a review of the literature. *American Journal of Kidney Diseases* 1993; **22** (suppl. 1: 23–31

A typically excellent Drugs review focusing on clinical data concerning the use of recombinant human Epo:
Faulds D, Sorkin EM. Epoetin (recombinant human erythropoietin): a review of its pharmacodynamic and pharmacokinetic properties and therapeutic potential in anaemia and the stimulation of erythropoiesis. *Drugs* 1989; **38**: 863–899

8

NADPH OXIDASE: ITS STRUCTURE AND ROLE

J. T. Hancock, P. J. Moulton and R. Desikan

SUMMARY

NADPH oxidase is a protein complex found in the plasma membrane of cells, the primary role of which is the production of the free radical superoxide. The enzyme normally resides in a quiescent state in which the membrane contains two polypeptides, which together constitute a heterodimeric flavocytochrome. On stimulation, several cytosolic polypeptides are translocated to the membrane to form the completed and active complex. These polypeptides include ones thought to be unique to NADPH oxidase as well as to the more generic signalling polypeptide, Rac. Dysfunction of NADPH oxidase components is the underlying cause of the condition of chronic granulomatous disease. This may be caused by the lack of a component, or the lack of the activity of a component, and therefore the disease has a complex genetic pattern and can in fact be inherited in both autosomal and X-linked fashions. Although originally thought to be unique to phagocytic cells, NADPH oxidase components have been found in many mammalian cells and recently in several plant species. It is now thought that NADPH oxidase might be involved in many cellular functions not only in the destructive role in which it was first implicated, but also as an oxygen sensor in some cells and as an integral part of cell signalling cascades in others.

INTRODUCTION

In 1933, Baldridge and Gerard reported that phagocytic cells showed an increase in oxygen consumption when stimulated, and it was thought that this was due to an increase in the respiration rate of the cells: the phenomenon was dubbed the 'respiratory burst'. However, in 1959, Sbarra and Karnovsky overturned the earlier view, and in 1961 Iyer et al showed that the increase in oxygen uptake was in fact also accompanied by an increase in the activity of the hexose monophosphate shunt (otherwise known as the pentose phosphate pathway) leading to the increased generation of NADPH. Today, it is known that the oxygen taken up during the respiratory burst is used for the generation of oxygen free radicals, catalysed by an enzyme complex known as NADPH oxidase.

The reaction catalysed by NADPH oxidase is the apparently simple transfer of a single electron, supplied originally by intracellular NADPH, to molecular oxygen producing a reactive superoxide ion ($O_2^{-\bullet}$):

$$2O_2 + NADPH \rightarrow 2O_2^{-\bullet} + NADP^+ + H^+.$$

The extra electron supplied to molecular oxygen is unpaired and therefore superoxide is classified as a free radical (denoted by the superscripted dot in chemical nomenclature). However, the pragmatic result is that the electronic state is relatively unstable and therefore superoxide is consequently comparatively reactive. One of the ways in which the superoxide ions can give up their extra electron is by undergoing what is known as a dismutation reaction. Here, two superoxide ions react together to produce hydrogen peroxide (H_2O_2):

$$2O_2^{-\bullet} + 2H^+ \rightarrow H_2O_2 + O_2.$$

While hydrogen peroxide is not strictly a free radical, it is commonly discussed with the oxygen free radicals. Many refer to oxygen-derived products under the umbrella term 'reactive oxygen species' (ROS) or 'active oxygen species' (AOS), and in many respects these might be better collective terms than 'oxygen free radicals' and *radical derived products.*

The reaction to form hydrogen peroxide will occur spontaneously, especially at low pH, but it is efficiently catalysed by superoxide dismutase (SOD). This enzyme has two main forms: a copper/zinc containing form ($Cu^{2+}/Zn^{2+}SOD$), which is found in the cytoplasm of cells, and a manganese-containing form, which is found in mitochondria.

Hydrogen peroxide produced by the above processes can also undergo further reactions. For example, superoxide and hydrogen peroxide react together with the formation of hydroxyl radicals ($OH^{\bullet}$):

$$O_2^{-\bullet} + H_2O_2 \rightarrow OH^{\bullet} + OH^- + O_2.$$

This reaction is particularly catalysed by the presence of free iron (Fe^{2+}) or copper (Cu^{2+}) ions.

Further reactive oxygen species can be formed enzymatically. Myeloperoxidase, found within the primary granules of neutrophils, catalyses the reaction:

$$H_2O_2 + Cl^- \rightarrow OCl^- + H^+ + OH^-.$$

Hypochlorous acid (OCl^-) is commonly used as a bleaching agent, and in a similar manner myeloperoxidase-derived hypochlorous acid is used as an antimicrobial agent by white blood cells.

Other reactive oxygen species that can be formed include singlet oxygen, which is also relatively unstable and reactive, and peroxynitrite ($OONO^-$), formed by the reaction of nitric oxide (generated by nitric oxide synthase) with superoxide:

$$NO^{\bullet} + O_2^{-\bullet} \rightarrow OONO^-.$$

Therefore a cascade of products can be formed initiated by the activity of NADPH oxidase. A quick glance at these products also reveals that many are very reactive, particularly hydroxyl radicals and hypochlorous acid, and it can therefore be seen how such activity may be harnessed by cells in a host-defence role.

A neutrophil chemotactic response results once a bacterium is sensed. This involves migration of the neutrophil towards the bacterium, and then the engulfment of the microbe by the formation of pseudopodia which wrap around it. The vacuole formed is known as a phagosome and comprises a bag of plasma membrane where the outside surface of the membrane faces the vacuole formed. Secretory vacuoles or granules in the neutrophil will then fuse with this phagosome membrane, and in doing so the contents of the granules are released inside the phagosome to come in direct contact with the bacterium. Several subgroups of granules have been identi- fied, but in general they all contain destructive enzymes such as proteases. However, of importance here, on formation of the phagocytic vacuole, NADPH oxidase activ- ity is initiated and superoxide and its resulting products are formed in the vicinity of the bacterium, causing damage, death and destruction of the microbe (Fig. 8.1).

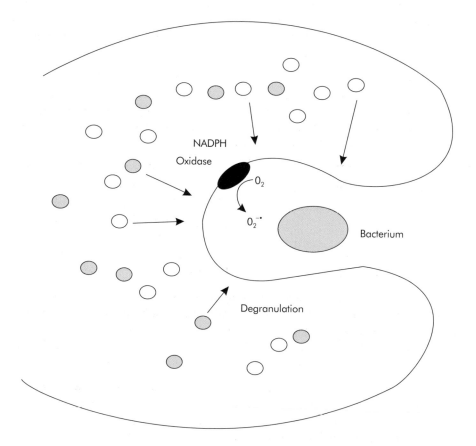

Figure 8.1 – Cellular events that occur when a bacterium is engulfed by a phagocytic cell.

Clear evidence of the importance of this activity is seen in chronic granulomatous disease (CGD) where activity of NADPH oxidase is impaired. A defective host-defence response is mounted by the neutrophils and commonly the individual suffers repeated infection, which if undetected will result in death at an early age. The molecular defects underlying this disease are discussed more fully below.

WHAT IS NADPH OXIDASE?

As noted above, the enzyme that facilitates the reduction of molecular oxygen to superoxide is NADPH oxidase. It has been well characterized primarily in phagocytic cell types particularly neutrophils. Although it has what appears to be a fairly simple task to perform – the single electron reduction of oxygen – a fair degree of complexity is associated with its structure and function. The reaction itself is thermodynamically relatively hard to achieve because the oxygen-to-superoxide redox couple has a very low mid-point potential. The end products of this enzyme-catalysed reaction (superoxide and its derived radicals) are highly toxic to both pathogen and host; thus, the functioning of NADPH oxidase has to be under tight regulation to ensure the enzyme is active only when necessary.

As the complexity of this enzyme is slowly being unravelled, there have been several conflicting opinions regarding the involvement of its various constituents. This review is intended to discuss current opinions regarding the structure of NADPH oxidase (Fig. 8.2), without going in to a detailed discussion of the experimentation from which they have been derived.

The electron transporter that carries electrons across the plasma membrane is a flavocytochrome complex. This is located primarily not only in the plasma membrane of neutrophils but also in their specific granules. The cytochrome is of a b-type, designated as either cytochrome b_{-245} or cytochrome b_{558}. The former refers to the low midpoint potential ($E_{m7.0} = -245mV$) of the cytochrome which has been shown to be sufficient for the reduction of O_2 to superoxide. The latter relates to the absorbance at 558nm of the α band of the cytochrome.

The cytochrome is a complex consisting of two subunits: a small subunit of approximately 22kDa, termed p22-*phox*, and a large β subunit of c.76–92kDa designated gp91-*phox*. (the term *phox* refers to phagocytic oxidase, and gp to glycosylated protein). In an intact NADPH oxidase system, this heterodimeric flavocytochrome consists of one molecule of each of the subunits.

The p22-*phox* mRNA transcript has been found to be present in many cell types but, interestingly, the protein is found only in cell types that also express gp91-*phox*. From studies in patients with CGD, and therefore deficient in the functioning of this respiratory burst oxidase, it appears that p22-*phox* and gp91-*phox* subunits are dependent on each other for stability.

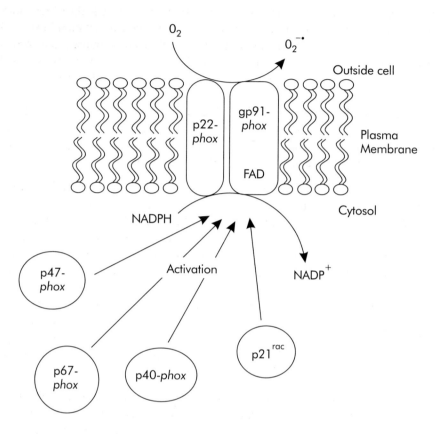

Figure 8.2 – A schematic representation of the NADPH oxidase complex.

As the NADPH oxidase protein complex is a cytochrome it must, by definition, contain a haem prosthetic group. The 22 kDa subunit was initially considered to be a candidate for the haem-bearing subunit of the cytochrome *b*, but it contains only one invariant histidine group which could partake in haem ligation. Furthermore, there have been recent suggestions that both the subunits share haem binding and that there are two haem groups present with slightly differing mid-point potentials – a fact that would make the nomenclature 'cytochrome b_{-245}' misleading! However, the exact nature of haem binding remains uncertain. A notable characteristic of the deduced primary amino acid sequence of p22-*phox* is that it has proline-rich target sequences in its C-terminal end: these have been implicated in interactions with other cytosolic subunits (see below).

The larger subunit of the cytochrome complex is the glycosylated protein designated as gp91-*phox*. Being heavily glycosylated, on SDS-PAGE this protein appears as a broad band between 76 and 92kDa. The N-terminal domain of the β subunit is hydrophobic with many membrane-spanning domains, while the C-terminus is more hydrophilic lying on the cytosolic side of the plasma membrane. This arrangement has a structural similarity to several electron transporting proteins from diverse origins including ferredoxin-NADP$^+$ reductases. gp91-*phox* is also believed to contain a FAD binding site, as well as a binding site for NADPH, the substrate for the activity of this enzyme. Thus, the cytochrome complex contains two important domains for the oxidoreductase activity: the flavin site as well as the haem centre, both of which act as electron transporters. Recent evidence also indicates that the cytosolic components of the enzyme complex participate in regulating electron flow between the various subunits (see below).

The functioning and activation of the NADPH enzyme complex is not complete without the involvement of several cytosolic proteins (Fig. 8.2). From studies in CGD patients, at least two of these proteins have been found to be critical to the functioning of the enzyme: 47 and 67 kDa termed p47-*phox* and p67-*phox* respectively. While the cell is in an inactive state, these proteins remain in the cytosol. Following activation, they translocate to the plasma membrane to be associated with the flavocytochrome *b* complex thus activating the enzyme. The interrelationship between these subunits for a functionally active enzyme is demonstrated by the observation that translocation of p67-*phox* does not occur in cells from CGD patients lacking p47-*phox*. In contrast, p47-*phox* does not depend on p67-*phox* for its translocation. There is also recent contradictory evidence suggesting that p47-*phox* is not essential for NADPH oxidase activity.

Interaction between the subunits of the NADPH oxidase occurs via specific protein-interaction domains. By binding to proline-rich domains on other proteins, Src homology 3 (SH3) domains are well-defined protein motifs that mediate protein–protein interactions in several eukaryotic signalling processes. Both the p47-*phox* and p67-*phox* proteins contain SH3 domains that enable interaction with one another and with the cytochrome. According to a current model, three SH3 domain interactions exist in the above mentioned proteins: one between p47-*phox* and the proline-rich region of p22-*phox* (cytochrome small subunit); the second and third interactions are between p47-*phox* and p67-*phox*, which promote their recruitment to the membrane. The involvement of another recently discovered protein with SH3 domains – the p40-*phox* – is discussed below.

Interestingly, both p47-*phox* and p67-*phox* appear to be phosphorylated following activation. This could lead to conformational changes in the proteins, facilitating their binding to the flavocytochrome. However, this phosphorylation does not seem to be a prerequisite for NADPH oxidase activity.

Apart from the structural importance of these proteins in mediating interactions between the cytochrome and cytosol, no definite function has been assigned to these cytosolic subunits. Only recently was it suggested that p47-*phox* and p67-*phox* might play roles in regulating the electron flow from NADPH to molecular oxygen. According to this hypothesis, p67-*phox* facilitates electron transfer between NADPH and FAD, while p47-*phox* is responsible for the movement of electrons from FAD, via the cytochrome *b* complex, to molecular oxygen. This view is supported by the discovery that p67-*phox* also possesses a NADPH binding site of higher affinity than the one said to be located on gp91-*phox*. Hence, as a result of activation when p67-*phox* is brought to the cytochrome, the two domains probably cooperate to form a single functionally active NADPH binding site, thus facilitating electron transfer. Again, there are conflicting views on these hypotheses, and the whole story regarding the function of these proteins is yet to be elucidated. Interestingly, no function has been found for these cytosolic proteins outside that of their interactions with the NADPH oxidase flavocytochrome, suggesting that they do have a definite and distinct role here and are not ubiquitous and generic signalling molecules.

The p40-*phox* protein (one of 40kDa) has recently been isolated and shown to bear an SH3 domain and to form part of the NADPH oxidase complex. In addition to the SH3 domain, p40-*phox* also contains a region that shows great similarity to the N-terminal region of p47-*phox*. In a cell-free system, p40-*phox* is not required for activity of NADPH oxidase. However, for enzyme functioning associated with the cytochrome, it requires the presence of both p47-*phox* and p67-*phox*. It has been hypothesized that p67-*phox* functions as a chaperone, to translocate p40-*phox* to the membrane following stimulation and where p40-*phox* could then bind to p47-*phox* via an SH3 domain. Very recently, it has been suggested that binding of the p40-*phox* component to p47-*phox* is in some way inhibitory to the functioning of the NADPH oxidase complex and is involved in its down-regulation. This opens a new and exciting possibility in the control of the release of free radicals by this complex.

Apart from these cytosolic proteins that comprise an active part of the NADPH oxidase, a group of small GTP-binding proteins have also been identified that appear to be essential to impart activity to the enzyme in an *in vitro* cell-free system. In the NADPH oxidase system, the complex consists of a *ras*-related protein p21[rac1] and the GDP-dissociation inhibitory factor (GDI). Activation of the complex is associated with p21[rac1] dissociating from GDI, GDP being exchanged for GTP on p21[rac1] and conversion of the Rac protein to its active form. Inactivation of the complex probably arises from GTP hydrolysis and a GTPase-activating protein (GAP), with p21[rac1] returning to its GDP-bound inactive state with GDI. The finding that superoxide acts as a signalling molecule spurred by a rac-mediated pathway adds a new dimension to the involvement of these molecules in signal transduction (discussed below).

ACTIVATION OF THE NADPH OXIDASE COMPLEX

The complexity of NADPH oxidase is not limited to its structural details. Unravelling the mechanism of activation of the oxidase has revealed that complex, and as yet not fully understood signal transduction pathways exist which lead to its activation.

NADPH oxidase in neutrophils can be activated, at least *in vitro*, by both receptor-dependent and -independent mechanisms. Stimulation via receptors can occur, for example, by the bacterial-related chemotactic peptide N-formyl-Met-Leu-Phe (FMLP) as well as by immune complexes. Alternatively, receptor-independent activation may occur through stimuli such as long chain-unsaturated fatty acids (arachidonic acid) and, less physiologically, by phorbol esters (PMA). Upon activation of neutrophils, the cytochrome *b*, the majority of which resides in granules located intracellularly, translocates to the plasma membrane in a process which requires continuous exposure of the cell to the stimulus. The oxidase is deactivated on removal of stimulus, but on second exposure it can be reactivated. Studies have revealed that the NADPH oxidase can be 'primed' by exposure to a sub-stimulatory dose of an activator. If, after a short period, the cells are exposed to a higher dose of the same or sometimes different stimuli, the subsequent response is both quicker (less lag time) and the free radical generation is greater.

It is currently thought that the signal transduction pathway leading to activation of NADPH oxidase (Fig. 8.3) is probably a membrane-bound receptor coupled to a heterotrimeric GTP-binding protein (G protein). Involvement of G proteins, such as the one referred to as G_q, may in turn lead to activation of phosphoinositol-specific phospholipase C (PLC), resulting in the breakdown of phosphatidylinositol 4,5-bisphosphate (PtdInsP$_2$) and increases in the intracellular

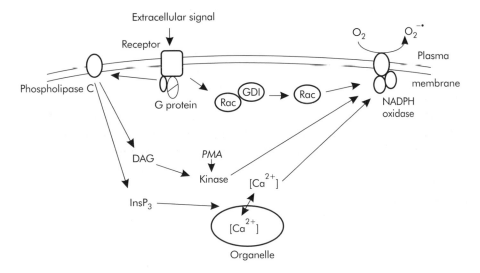

Figure 8.3 – Possible intracellular signalling pathways that might lead to activation of NADPH oxidase.

concentrations of both diacylglycerol (DAG) and inositol trisphosphate (InsP$_3$). This would lead to release of intracellular calcium ions and activation of protein kinase C, both of which are known to activate the NADPH oxidase.

An increase in levels of intracellular Ca^{2+} results in translocation of the cytosolic components of the oxidase to the plasma membrane and hence an increased respiratory burst activity. However, the addition of Ca^{2+} ionophores such as ionomycin or A23187 does not appear to be sufficient for full respiratory burst activity. Furthermore, by diminishing the levels of intracellular Ca^{2+} by the use of Ca^{2+} chelators, enhancement of the respiratory burst is not impaired, suggesting that factors other than Ca^{2+} partake in activation of the enzyme complex.

As well as the involvement of calcium ions it is also believed that phosphorylation is critical for the activation of NADPH oxidase. The phorbol ester phorbol 12-myristate 13-acetate (PMA) is a structural analogue of DAG, a molecule which activates protein kinase C (PKC). In fact, PMA is routinely used in the laboratory to activate neutrophil free radical release. Such activation of NADPH oxidase is prolonged by the addition of a phosphatase inhibitor such as okadaic acid, thus emphasizing the role of phosphorylation in the activation of the oxidase. Activation of the oxidase by PMA can occur in the absence of increased intracellular Ca^{2+} concentrations thereby strengthening the above hypothesis that calcium-dependent and calcium-independent pathways exist. Although the exact identity of the kinase involved is not known, it has been shown that PMA activates PKC, and that the cytochrome *b* and cytosolic components (p47-*phox* and p67-*phox*) become phosphorylated following activation. Phosphorylation may result in the change in conformation of proteins, which could then allow interaction via SH3 domains between the various subunits to form an activated complex. However, as stated above, phosphorylation of the cytosolic NADPH oxidase components is not crucial to stimulation of free radical generation.

Taken together, the results suggest that several pathways may lead to the activation of the oxidase, and an interplay between these diverging and converging pathways leads to the ultimate stimulation of NADPH oxidase activity. Recent work with inhibitors such as the fungal compound wortmannin, which inhibits phosphorylation of membrane lipids, suggests that pathways as yet to be elucidated are probably also involved.

As noted above, activation of NADPH oxidase results in the extracellular production of superoxide and the transfer of electrons (negative charge) across plasma membranes. This generates, therefore, a differential charge across the membrane, which needs to be dispersed or the oxidase will stop functioning. There are some conflicting views regarding expulsion of protons across the plasma membrane to neutralize the negative charge, but it has been suggested that protons are moved as compensatory ions through a proton channel which opens when the NADPH oxidase is activated. This could result in a decrease in pH of phagocytic vacuoles which, along with the release of granule contents into the lumen of the vacuole, facilitates the killing of invading microbes. In fact, the exact mechanisms by which the invading microbes are killed in the phagocytic vacuole remain to be elucidated, but some data suggest that the role of the free radicals is limited with alterations in pH being crucial: indeed, the change of pH might be a primary function of NADPH oxidase activity.

CHRONIC GRANULOMATOUS DISEASE

The importance of an active NADPH oxidase complex in the fight against pathogenic invasion is highlighted by CGD. The disease manifests itself as a recurrent series of bacterial and fungal infections, leading to granulomatous infiltration of major organs, and if left untreated an early death. These infections commonly involve *Staphylococci* spp., *Serratia marcescens*, *Klebsiella* spp., *Aerobacter* spp., *Salmonella* spp., *Aspergillus* spp., *Candida* spp. or *Nocardia* spp.

Recent molecular biology techniques have revealed that all cases of CGD are due to lack of a functioning NADPH oxidase. Early work was confused, as reports that appeared in the literature stated that the disease was inherited in both an autosomal and X-linked fashion. However, as can be seen from Table 8.1, both scenarios are possible with the lack of NADPH oxidase activity being attributable to a lack or dysfunction in any one of four of the NADPH oxidase components – gp91-*phox*, p22-*phox*, p47-*phox* and p67-*phox*. No case of the disease has been reported due to a defect of either p40-*phox* or the G protein activator p21^{rac}, although the lack of function of the latter would probably have profound effects on the cell.

Table 8.1 – Classification and modes of inheritance defined for chronic granulomatous disease.

Mode of inheritance	Subtype	NAPDH oxidase component involved	% of cases (approx.)
X-linked	X91^{0}	gp-91-*phox*	50
	X91^{-}		3
	X91^{+}		3
Autosomal	A22^{0}	p22-*phox*	5
	A22^{+}		1
Autosomal	A47^{0}	p47-*phox*	33
Autosomal	A67^{0}	p67-*phox*	5

In descriptions of the subtypes of chronic granulomatous disease, the first letter of the subtype denotes the inheritance pattern where X=X-linked and A=autosomal. Superscripts denote whether the component is completely undetectable (^{0}), diminished in amount ($^{-}$) or present in normal amounts but dysfunctional ($^{+}$).

Approximately 50% of CGD cases are associated with a complete lack of the gp91-*phox* component and are inherited in an X-linked fashion. Interestingly, in this form of the disease the p22-*phox* protein is also missing: it is presumably produced by the cell but, because no stable complex can be formed, it is destroyed and therefore remains undetected. However, other forms of X-linked CGD include situations where the gp91-*phox* component is reduced or, if present, is apparently non-functional. For example, the lack of activity of gp91-*phox* might be due to a single-point mutation within the relevant gene (*CYBB*). However, other mutations reported include small deletions, nonsense and missense mutations, splice site defects leading to poor processing of the mRNA, and mutations within the regulatory region of the gene.

The most common form of autosomal CGD is caused by a defect in the cytosolic component, p47-*phox*. A common defect found here is a dinucleotide deletion from the the *NCF1* gene. Other forms of autosomal disease include deletions, missense mutations and frameshifts within the p22-*phox* gene (*CYTA*). Interestingly, in forms of CGD that show a lack of the p67-*phox* gene product, the p40-*phox* protein is also seen to be reduced in amount.

Now that the genes that code for the NADPH oxidase components have been cloned, sequenced and fairly well characterized, there is optimism that a long and lasting cure for CGD may be possible with somatic gene therapy techniques. In these techniques, the appropriate 'good' gene is targetted, perhaps to the bone marrow, where even only a low percentage of NADPH oxidase activity would result in significant clinical benefit.

NADPH OXIDASE IN NON-PHAGOCYTIC SYSTEMS

NADPH oxidase in other mammalian cells

A phagocyte-like NADPH oxidase has been reported in a number of different cell types from both human and other mammalian sources, including cells such as fibroblasts, kidney mesangial cells, chondrocytes from cartilage, endothelial cells, aortic smooth muscle cells and carotid body type I cells. Although identified using either antibodies raised against human phagocytic NADPH oxidase components or by the use of polymerase chain reaction (PCR) primers against published human phagocytic cell NADPH oxidase mRNA sequences, the NADPH oxidase complexes identified in these other cell types have yet to be fully characterized. However, it has been suggested that NADPH oxidase exists as isoforms in these non-phagocytic cell types, although at present there is only circumstantial evidence to support this theory. For example, fibroblasts from CGD patients may contain a fully functional NADPH oxidase, which might suggest that fibroblast and neutrophil NADPH oxidase are both structurally and genetically distinct. Other evidence to support the isoenzyme theory comes from immunological studies of the cytochrome *b* (gp91-*phox*) component from various cell types, different levels of NADPH oxidase activity in various cell types and differences in the stimulation, suppression and inhibition of NADPH oxidase.

Plant NADPH oxidase

The distribution of NADPH oxidase is not limited to the animal kingdom. In plants, there is evidence to suggest that a plasma membrane-bound NADPH oxidase-like enzyme exists, which as in animals serves a role in pathogen defence. The rationale for this theory is that when plants are invaded by potential pathogens, an oxidative or respiratory burst occurs and the ROS formed help to limit pathogen growth and potentiate localized cell death in the host – in a manner analogous to programmed cell death in animals.

Data derived from immunological studies suggest that both soybean and *Arabidopsis thaliana* contain components related to the p22-*phox*, p47-*phox* and p67-*phox* proteins of the NADPH oxidase complex. Recently, a rice homologue of gp91-*phox* has been cloned thus further supporting the possibility of plant-associated NADPH oxidase. Further characterization of the NADPH oxidase in plants is likely to reveal the evolutionary significance of this enzyme complex.

ROLES OF REACTIVE OXYGEN SPECIES GENERATED BY NADPH OXIDASE
Destructive roles

The primary role of NADPH oxidase is the production of superoxide which, as outlined above, undergoes subsequent reactions to form other ROS occurring during the neutrophil respiratory burst. Such activity is thought to be involved directly in the destruction of foreign matter, including pathogens, that has entered the body. Both superoxide and hydrogen peroxide are relatively non-destructive and have short half-lives. Hydrogen peroxide is only a weak oxidizing agent and is efficiently removed by catalase or the glutathione cycle. Potentially more destructive than either superoxide or hydrogen peroxide are hydroxyl radicals that oxidize proteins and lipids, and cause damage to DNA; singlet oxygen has been shown to destroy carotenes, haem proteins and membrane lipids. Hypochlorite and peroxynitrite are the two ROS that are most destructive. Both are strong oxidizing agents and are probably responsible for the majority of damage done to invading cells that have been phagocytosed.

ROS also have a less direct destructive potential due to their ability to stimulate the production of, or to modify, other degradative enzymes. For example, ROS have been implicated in the onset and development of inflammatory joint diseases including rheumatoid arthritis and osteoarthritis. It has been demonstrated that hydrogen peroxide converts pro-collagenases to active forms of the enzyme that are probably involved in the destruction of the cartilage matrix. However, all the activities of ROS are not destructive. At low concentrations, they may stimulate cell proliferation and production of structural proteins such as proteoglycans (see below).

Potential signalling role of ROS

The possibility that ROS could function as signalling molecules was first suggested when it was realised that NADPH oxidase appears to be present in many cell types but levels of superoxide production by non-phagocytic cell types are too low for it to have any destructive role. Furthermore, release of ROS by non-phagocytic cells was over a much longer time scale (hours in some cases), and constitutive production of ROS in some cells has also been reported.

On the basis that it seems a waste of cellular resources to retain the ability to express non-essential genes in a differentiated cell type, it has been assumed that NADPH oxidase and the superoxide it produces must be essential for some cellular function(s). While ROS may promote the synthesis of some proteins (see above), it has also been demonstrated that ROS are involved in the regulation of a number of key molecules involved in intracellular signalling: hydrogen peroxide and, to a lesser extent, nitric oxide both stimulate *c-jun* NH_2-terminal kinase activity thus increasing the expression of *c-jun*, the protein product of which combines with the protein product of *c-fos* to form the transcriptional regulator AP-1. Other intracellular signalling roles proposed for ROS (particularly hydrogen peroxide) include activation of the transcription factor NF-κB probably through dissociation from its inhibitor protein I-κB. Such a scheme is illustrated in Fig. 8.4, where activation by the monomeric G protein Rac stimulates NADPH oxidase to produce superoxide ions, the dismutation of which to hydrogen peroxide might lead to the activation of NF-kB and thus alterations in nuclear gene expression.

Other signalling roles for ROS include activation of MAP kinase pathways and guanylyl cyclase. It is possible that low concentrations of ROS are vital signals that control the synthesis of new proteins in a wide variety of physiological situations. Clearly more work is required to reveal the exact mechanisms.

Oxygen sensing by a NADPH oxidase-like complex

The presence of a phagocyte-like NADPH oxidase complex has been described in a number of cell types implicated in oxygen homeostasis. These include human carotid body type I cells, neuroepithelial bodies of the lung and erythropoietin-producing HepG2 cells. Two pieces of evidence suggest the involvement of NADPH oxidase in oxygen sensing in the carotid body:

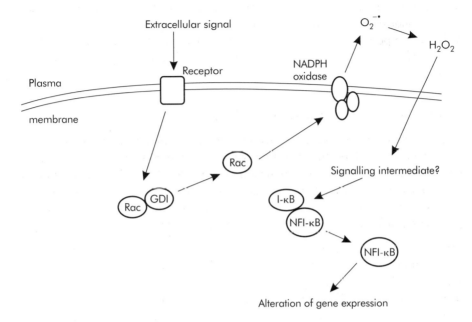

Figure 8.4 – A possible signalling cascade in which NADPH oxidase is integral. Hydrogen peroxide, generated by the dismutation of superoxide, may result in activation of the transcription factor NF-κB and therefore may control the level of expression of specific genes.

- generation of hydrogen peroxide is an essential step in the events that link hypoxia to the stimulation of nerve endings; and

- the pO_2 value of neutrophil NADPH oxidase (7 Torr) is within the range suitable for monitoring pO_2 in the carotid body under hypoxia.

Recent papers suggest that the hydrogen peroxide produced as a result of NADPH oxidase activity in such cells is used to control the functioning of a K^+-channel in the plasma membranes. However, whether the NADPH oxidase is the same as that found in phagocytic cells or is an isoenzyme form needs to be elucidated.

CONCLUSIONS

It is now clear that superoxide and the resulting free radicals are produced by many phagocytic cells, and that the main enzyme involved in this activity is the NADPH oxidase complex. The molecular biology of this complex is slowly being unravelled and almost certainly will be a target for somatic gene therapy in the search for a cure for chronic granulomatous disease. However, what is also becoming increasingly clear is the fact that this enzyme exists in many non-phago-cytic cells, and it even appears in plant tissue. Undoubtedly, one of the main challenges now is to identify roles for the enzyme and its products in these tissues. We need to understand how the production of relatively destructive compounds such as hydrogen peroxide can fit into cell signalling cascades, to understand how such activity is regulated and its interplay with other systems, such as those involving nitric oxide, so that we can get a better comprehension of the role of NADPH oxidase in the control of cellular function.

SELECTED READING FOR MORE DETAILED INFORMATION

A recent review of the production and role of oxygen-free radicals, including nitric oxide, but it does not include the most recent ras cascades published in Science (see below):
Hancock JT. Superoxide, hydrogen peroxide and nitric oxide as signalling molecules: their production and role in disease. *British Journal of Biomedical Sciences* 1997; **54**: 38–46

A relatively recent review of the phagocytic NADPH oxidase, but it has a strong bias towards the movement of protons which is thought to accompany the release of superoxide by the NADPH oxidase complex:
Henderson LM, Chappell JB. NADPH oxidase of neutrophils. *Biochimica Biophysica Acta* 1996; **1273**: 87–107

An excellent paper on the role of oxygen-free radicals in cell signalling cascades:
Irani K, Xia Y, Zweier JL et al. Mitogenic signaling mediated by oxidants in *ras* transformed fibroblasts. *Science* 1997l **275**: 1649–1651

One of a number of recent reviews on the molecular biology of chronic granulomatous disease. Other mutations have been identified since the publication of this review, but the principles have remained the same:
Pallister CJ, Hancock JT. Phagocytic NADPH oxidase and its role in chronic granulomatous disease. *British Journal of Biomedical Sciences* 1995; **52**: 149–156

An excellent and up-to-date summary of the role of oxygen radicals in the response of plants to pathogen attack, including a discussion of the plant NADPH oxidase:
Wojtaszek P. Oxidative burst: an early plant response to pathogen infection. *Biochemical Journal* 1997; **322**: 681–692

A recent paper showing a potential signalling pathway involving oxygen-free radicals, where NADPH oxidase is acting as an oxygen sensor, clearly in an area in which there will be more interest:
Wang D, Youngson C, Yeger H et al. NADPH oxidase and a hydrogen peroxide sensitive K+ channel may function as an oxygen sensor complex in airway chemoreceptors and small cell lung carcinoma cell lines. *Proceedings of the National Academy of Sciences, USA* 1996; **93**: 13182–13187

INDEX

5q-syndrome, 89

Acquired immune deficiency syndrome
    (AIDS), 57
Acquisition, 41–42
Acute lymphoblastic leukaemia (ALL),
    19–23
  B cell (Burkitt's), 19, 20, 21, 50, 51
  biophenotypic, 20
  classifications, 30–31
  cytogenetic classification, 20–21, 22
  drug resistance, 22–23
  FAB classification, 19, 23
  flow karyotyping, 59
  immunophenotypic classification, 19–20,
    22
  leukaemogenesis, 50
  M3, 52
  molecular classification, 21, 22
  morphological classification, 19, 22
  null ALL, 19, 20
  phenotypic analysis, 50
  Philadelphia chromosome, 20–21
  precursor B cell, 19, 20, 51
  precursor T cell, 20
  prognosis, 51
  scoring systems, 22
  T cell, 19, 50
Acute myelocytic leukaemia (AML),
    24–26
  congenital, 26
  Down's syndrome, 26
  FAB classification, 24–25
  flow karyotyping, 59

M0, 24, 51
M1, 24
M2, 24
M3 (promyelocytic), 24–25
M4 (myelomonocytic), 24
M5 (monoblastic/monocytic), 24, 51
M6 (erythroleukaemia), 24, 26, 51
M7 (megakaryoblastic), 24, 51
  myelodysplastic syndromes, 30
  phenotypic analysis, 50–51
Adult T cell leukaemia, 47
Aerobacter spp., 165
Agrobacterium tumefaciens, 140
ALL-*trans*-retinoic acid (ATRA), 25, 52
Alopecia, 6
Amplification, 42
Anaemia
  hypoplastic, 30
  aplastic, 10, 11
1-Antichymotrypsin, 76
Antibody binding quantification, 44–45
Anti-glycophorin-A, 51
Antimyeloperoxidase (anti-MPO), 50–51
Anti-proliferation bioassays, 76
Antithymocyte globulin, 8, 9
Anti-viral assays, 76
Apheresis, 3
Aplastic anaemia, 10, 11
Apoptosis, 115, 118, 126
Aspergillus infections, 9, 165
Autoimmune neutropaenia (AIN), 57
Autoimmune thrombocytopaenia (ATP),
    56
axl gene, 98

B cell acute lymphoblastic leukaemia (B ALL), 19, 20, 21, 50, 51
B cell chronic lymphocytic leukaemia (B CLL), 27–29
B cell prolymphocytic leukaemia (B PLL), 54
B cells
  antigen affinity, 106
  bone marrow, 106–107
  CD5+, 116–117
  circulating antigen, 117–118
  development, 105, 106–118
  DNA rearrangements, 107–117
  growth factors, 99, 100
  immune reconstitution, 8
  immunoglobulin class switching, 118
  phenotypic changes, 116
  potentially autoreactive, 115–116
  receptor editing, 115
  repertoire, 106
Bacillus subtilis, 141
Bernard Soulier syndrome (BSS), 56
Beta-TG, 71
Bone marrow
  B cell development, 106–107
  chimeras, 121–123
  colony-forming assays, 67, 77
  harvest, 3
  T cell development, 121–123
  transplantation, 57
Breast cancer, 10
Bronchiolitis obliterans, 8
Busulphan, 6

Calcium, 78
Candida infections, 9, 165
Cataracts, 9
CD1, 126
CD2, 50, 53, 100, 126
CD3, 43, 49, 123, 125, 126, 129
CD4+ T cells
  distribution, 46
  immune recognition, 5
  recovery after bone marrow transplantation, 57
CD4+/CD8+ ratio, 46
CD5, 116–117, 126

CD7, 51, 53, 125, 126
CD8+ T cells
  distribution, 46
  immune recognition, 5
  recovery after bone marrow transplantation, 57
CD10, 50, 116
CD11b, 51, 53
CD13, 50–51, 53
CD14 (lipopolysaccharide receptor), 43, 51, 56
CD15, 51
CD16, 43, 56
CD19, 50, 53, 116
CD20, 116
CD21, 116
CD22, 43, 116
CD23, 76, 116
CD25, 125
CD27, 98
CD28, 100
CD30, 98
CD33, 50–51, 53
CD34, 4, 125
CD34-enriched blast cell colony-forming (BCCF) assay, 98
CD38, 116, 126
CD40, 98, 116
CD41, 51
CD42, 51
CD44, 125
CD45
  antigen, 43
  receptor, 116
CD55 (decay accelerating factor), 56
CD61, 51
CD68, 51
CD71, 126
CD72, 116
CD117 (kit receptor), 106
Cell adhesion molecules, 106, 121
Cell-line based assays, 70
Cell sorting, 45
  acute leukaemias, 51–52
Cell surface molecules, 76
c-fms, 97
CFU-E, 145

CFU–GEMM, 99
Chemokine family, 92
Chemotaxis assays, 77–78
Chlorambucil, 54
Chlorodeoxyadenosine, 54
Chromosomes
    abnormalities, 59–60
    immunoglobulin gene segments,
        107–108
    sorting, 51–52
Chronic eosinophilic leukaemia, 27
Chronic granulocytic leukaemia (CGL),
    26–27, 56
Chronic granulomatous disease (CGD),
    159, 161, 165–166
Chronic lymphocytic leukaemia (CLL),
    27–29
    FAB classification, 27–28
    phenotypic analysis, 54
    scoring system, 54
Chronic myelocytic leukaemia (CML),
    26–27, 56
    atypical, 27
    FAB classification, 26–27
Chronic myelomonocytic leukaemia
    (CMML), 27, 30
Chronic neutrophilic leukaemia, 27
c-kit, 97
Cladribine, 29
Clusters of differentiation (CD), 42
Cosmids, 52
Cyanine-5, 43
CyChrome, 43
Cyclophosphamide, 6, 57
Cyclosporin, 2, 8
Cytokines, 63–86
    antiproliferation bioassays, 76
    anti-viral assays, 77
    assays, 67–80
    bioassays, 67–78
    bone marrow colony-forming assays, 77
    cell surface molecule assays, 76
    chemotaxis assays, 77–78
    cytotoxic assays, 77
    detection in cells/tissues, 80–81
    glycosylation, 66
    immunoassays, 78–79

inhibition assays, 77
ionic flux measurement, 78
kinase receptor activation assay (KIRA),
    78
mRNA expression, 81
production, 67
proliferation bioassays, 76
properties, 64–66
receptor binding assays, 80
reporter gene-based assays, 78
respiratory burst assays, 78
sample preparation, 81–82
secondary molecule secretion, 76
standardization, 82–84
statistical evaluation, 82–84
Cytomegalovirus, 9
Cytotoxic assays, 77

Decay accelerating factor (DAF, CD55), 56
Deep vein thrombosis, 58
Dendritic cells, 60, 121, 125
Deoxycoformycin, 54
Diamorphine, 6
DiGeorge syndrome, 119
Dihydrofolate reductase (DHFR), 149
Dimethylsulphoxide, 4
DNA
    B cell development, 107–117
    dual-immunofluorescence, 43
    erythropoietin production, 136–142,
        146–150
    index, 21
    polymerase chain reaction, 52
Donor-cell leukaemia, 9, 12
Donor leucocyte infusion (DLI), 12
Down's syndrome, 26
Dual-immunofluorescence, 43
EBV-associated lymphoproliferative
    disease, 9, 12
EGF receptor, 96
Elastase, 76
ENA-78 bioassays, 71
Encephalomyocarditis virus, 77
Enzyme-linked immunosorbent assays
    (ELISAs), 78–79
Enzyme-linked immunospot (ELISPOT)
    procedure, 80–81

Eph-like receptors, 97
Epidermal growth factor (EGF)
  family, 92
  receptor, 96
erbB-2 receptor, 96
Erythrocytes, 4
Erythroleukaemia, 24, 26, 51
Erythropoietin (EPO), 91, 99
  activity, 64
  bioassays, 70
  cell line-based assays, 74
  clinical uses, 150–151
  commercial production, 141–142
  glycosylation, 66
  in vitro gene expression, 140–141
  post-hypoxic polycythaemic mouse
    assay, 67
  production, 143–145, 146–150
  receptors, 93, 94, 146
  recombinant DNA technology, 136–142,
    146–150
  regulation of erythropoiesis, 142–143
  secretion, 89
  site of action, 145–146
  therapeutic, 67
Escherichia coli, 137–139, 141, 149
Essential thrombasthemia, 58
Ethanol, 43

FACSCalibur Sort, 45
FAS, 98
Fibroblast growth factor family, 91
Fibroblast growth factor receptor family, 97
Ficoll-Hypaque density gradient
    centrifugation, 46
Flavocytochrome, 159, 161–162
Flow cytometry, 35–62
  cell function analysis, 58
  cell sorting, 45
  chromosome sorting, 51–52
  diagnostic applications, 45–60
  flow karyotyping, 59–60
  history/development, 36
  laser-based, 40
  light scatter/detection, 40
  minimal residual disease detection,
    58–60

principles, 37–45
  rare event analysis, 58
Flow karyotyping, 59–60
Flt-1, 97
Flt-3 ligand, 13
  bioassays, 69
Fludarabine, 29
Fluorescein isothiocyanate (FITC), 43
Fluorescence analysis, 41
Fluorescence quantification, 43–44
Fluorescence relative channel number
    (RCN), 44
Fluorochrome:protein ratio, 44
Follicular dendritic cells, 118
Follicular lymphoma, 27, 54
Forward angle light (FAL) sensors, 40

Gastrointestinal tract, 7
GATA-1, 145
G-CSF, 57, 58, 66, 91, 98, 99, 107
  bioassays, 69
  bone marrow colony-formation assays,
    77
  cell line-based assays, 73
  receptor, 93, 94
  therapeutic, 67
GDP-dissociation inhibitory factor (GDI),
    162
Germ cell tumours, 10
Glanzmann's thrombasthaemia (GT), 56
Beta-Glucuronidase, 76
Glycoproteins, 56
GM-CSF, 57, 58, 66, 91, 99, 107
  bioassays, 69, 76
  bone marrow colony-formation assays,
    77
  cell line-based assays, 73
  IFN-mediated inhibition, 77
  receptor, 93, 94
  therapeutic, 67
gp10, 91
gp91-*phox*, 159–161, 165–166, 167
gp130 subunit, 94, 95
G-protein coupled receptors, 98
G-proteins, 92, 153
Graft versus host disease (GVHD), 2, 4, 5,
    7–8

Graft versus tumour effect, 11
Granulocyte infusions, 9
Granulocyte-macrophage colony-forming unit (CFU-GM) assay, 4
GRO-MGSA
  bioassays, 71
  cell line-based assays, 75
Growth disorders, 9
Growth factors, 87–101
  B cells, 99, 100
  functions, 98 100
  genes, structure/expression, 89–90
  groups (1–4), 91–92
  lineage-specific, 99
  molecular genetics, 89–100
  mRNA, 89–90
  nomenclature, 88–89
  pleiotropy, 89
  receptors, 93–98
  redundancy, 89
  structural classification, 90–93

Haematopoietic growth factors *see* Growth factors
Haematopoietic stem cells, 104
  transplantation *see* Stem cell transplantation
Haematopoietin
  domains, 91, 92
  receptors, 93–95
Hairy cell leukaemia, 27, 54
Hashimoto's disease, 47
Helper T cells, 57
Heparin, 82
Hepatocyte growth factor receptor (HGF-R; scatter factor), 97
Herpes simplex infection, 9
Herpes zoster infection, 9
Hexose monophosphate shunt (pentose phosphate pathway), 156
Hickmann lines, infection, 8
High proliferative potential colony-forming cell (HPP-CFC) assay, 98–99
Histograms, 42
Homogeneously staining regions (HSRs), 52
HTLV-1 positive T cell lymphomas, 47

Human leucocyte antigens (HLA), 5
4-Hydroperoxycyclophosphamide, 4
Hydrogen peroxide, 157, 167, 168–169
Hypochlorite, 167
Hypochlorous acid, 157
Hypothyroidism, 9
Hypoxia, 142–145

I-309 bioassays, 71
ICAM-1, 76
Iccosomes, 118
IgA, 100
IgD
  B cell development, 115, 116, 118
  receptors, 107
IgG, 100
IgM, 43, 100
  B cell development, 109–110, 115, 116, 118
  leukaemia diagnosis, 49
  receptors, 107
Immune status
  correlation with disease course, 57–58
  following therapy, 57–58
  immune reconstitution, 8
  initial assessment, 45–47
Immunofluorescence, 43
Immunoglobulins
  chromosomal arrangements, 107–108
  class switching, 118
  growth factors, 100
  see also IgA; IgD; IgG; IgM
Immunophenotyping, 47
Immunoradiometric assays (IRMAs), 78–79
Immunosuppression, 5–6
In situ hybridization, 52, 60, 81
Infantile monosomy 7 syndrome, 27
Infection, 8–9, 14
Inflammatory joint diseases, 167
Insulin receptor, 96
Insulin-like growth factor (IGF) receptor, 96
Insulin-related growth factor family, 92
Interferon-alpha (IFN-alpha), 54
  cell line-based assays, 74
  chronic myeloid leukaemia, 27
  therapeutic, 67

Interferon-beta (IFN-beta)
 cell line-based assays, 75
 therapeutic, 67
Interferon-gamma (IFN-gamma), 66, 91,
 100
 cell line-based assays, 75
 cell surface molecules, 76
 ELISPOT, 80
Interleukin 1 (IL-1), 91, 99, 100, 107
 activity, 64, 66
 bioassays, 68
 cell line-based assays, 72
 IL-2 secretion, 76
 pyrogen assay, 67
Interleukin 1-alpha (IL-1-alpha), 66
 cell surface molecules, 76
 immunoassays, 78
Interleukin 1-beta (IL-1-beta), 66
 cell surface molecules, 76
 immunoassays, 78
Interleukin 2 (IL-2), 66, 91, 99, 100
 bioassays, 68
  cell line-based assays, 72, 76
 receptor, 93, 95, 99–100
 T cell development, 121
 therapeutic, 67
 WHO International Standard, 82
Interleukin 3 (IL-3), 66, 91, 98–99
 bioassays, 68
 bone marrow colony-formation assays,
 77
 cell line-based assays, 72
 production, 64
 receptor, 93, 94, 106–107
Interleukin 4 (IL-4), 66, 91, 98, 99, 100
 B cell development, 106
 bioassays, 68
 cell line-based assays, 72, 76
 cell surface molecules, 76
 receptor, 93, 94, 95
Interleukin 5 (IL-5), 91, 99, 100
 activity, 64
 bioassays, 68
 cell line-based assays, 72
 receptor, 93, 94
 TGFb-mediated inhibition, 77
Interleukin 6 (IL-6), 66, 91, 98, 99, 100

 activity, 64
 bioassays, 68
 cell line-based assays, 72
 ELISPOT, 80
 IgG secretion, 76
 receptor, 93, 94, 95
 sample preparation, 82
Interleukin 7 (IL-7), 91, 99, 100
 B cell development, 106
 bioassays, 68
 cell line-based assays, 72
 receptor, 93, 95
 T cell development, 121
Interleukin 8 (IL-8), 92
 bioassays, 71, 76
 receptor, 98
 respiratory burst assays, 78
Interleukin 9 (IL-9), 91
 bioassays, 68
 cell line-based assays, 73
 receptor, 93, 95
Interleukin 10 (IL-10), 91
 bioassays, 68
 cell line-based assays, 73
 ELISPOT, 80
 IFN-gamma inhibition, 76
Interleukin 11 (IL-11), 91
 bioassays, 68
 cell line-based assays, 73
 receptor, 93, 95
Interleukin 12 (IL-12), 66, 91, 92
 bioassays, 69
 cell line-based assays, 73
Interleukin 13 (IL-13), 91
 bioassays, 69
 cell line-based assays, 73
Interleukin 14 (IL-14), 69
Interleukin 15 (IL-15)
 bioassays, 69
 cell line-based assays, 73
 receptor, 93, 95
Interleukin 16 (IL-16), 69
Interleukin 17 (IL-17), 69
Interleukin 18 (IL-18), 69
Intestinal intraepithelial lymphocytes
 (IEL), 131–132
IP-10 bioassays, 71

Janus kinase (Jak-2), 93, 95
Juvenile chronic myelomonocytic
    leukaemia (JCML), 27

KD-R, 97
Kinase receptor activation assay (KIRA),
    78
kit
    receptor (CD117), 106
    T cell development, 121
Klebsiella spp., 165

Large cell lymphomas, 54
Large granular lymphocytes, 57
Large granular lymphocytic leukaemia
    (LGL), 55
Leucopheresis, 3
Leukaemias, 17–33
    acute lymphoblastic *see* Acute
        lymphoblastic leukaemia
    acute myelocytic *see* Acute myelocytic
        leukaemia
    acute promyelocytic, 25
    adult T cell, 47
    B cell chronic lymphocytic, 27–29
    biphenotypic acute, analysis, 53
    blast cell differentiation, 48–49
    cell sorting, 51–52
    chromosome abnormalities, 51–52
    chronic eosinophilic, 27
    chronic granulocytic, 26–27, 56
    chronic lymphocytic *see* Chronic
        lymphocytic leukaemia
    chronic myelocytic *see* Chronic
        myelocytic leukaemia
    chronic myelomonocytic, 27, 30
    chronic neutrophilic, 27
    classification, 18–19, 30–31, 48
    congenital, 26
    diagnosis, 48–57
    DNA index, 21
    donor-cell, 9, 12
    donor leucocyte infusion, 12
    hairy cell, 27, 54
    immunophenotypic analysis, 48–49
    juvenile chronic myelomonocytic, 27
    large granular lymphocytic (LGL), 55

morphology, immunology, cytogentic
    (MIC) scheme, 51
prolymphocytic, 27, 55
relapse, 58–60
stem cell transplantation, 4, 10
T cell, 55
translocations, 51–52
Leukocyte inhibitory factor (LIF), 91
    bioassays, 70
    cell line-based assays, 74
    receptor, 93, 95
Lipopolysaccharide, 90
    receptor (CD14), 43, 51, 56
Liver, 7
Long-term culture-initiating cells
    (LTCIC), 13
Luciferase, 78
Lymphocytes, 104
    dual-positive CD4+,CD8+, 47
    gating, 46
    intestinal intraepithelial, 131–132
    recovery after bone marrow
        transplantation, 57
    subsets, 45–47
    see also B cells; T cells
Lymphomas
    follicular, 27, 54
    HTLV-1 positive T cell, 47
    immunophenotypic analysis, 48–49
    large cell, 54
    mantle cell, 27, 54
    non-Hodgkin's, 10, 54
    splenic lymphoma with villous
        lymphocytes (SLVL), 27, 54
    stem cell transplantation, 4
    T cell, 55
Lymphopenia, 8
Lymphoproliferative diseases, 27–29
    EBV-associated, 9, 12
    phenotypic analysis, 54–55
Lysolecithin, 43

Mafosfamide, 4
Major histocompatibility complex (MHC), 5
    T cell development, 118–119, 128–130
Mantle cell lymphoma, 27, 54
MAP kinase pathway, 95

MCP-1,-2,-3, 92, 98
  bioassays, 71
  cell line-based assays, 75
M-CSF, 66, 91, 99, 107
  activity, 64
  bioassays, 69
  bone marrow colony-formation assays, 77
  cell line-based assays, 73
  receptor, 97
Megakaryocyte growth and differentiation factor, 13
Methotrexate, 2
Minimal residual disease, 58–60
MIP-1-alpha, 92, 98
  bioassays, 71
  cell line-based assays, 75
MIP-1-beta, 92, 98
  bioassays, 71
MIP-2, 92, 98
Molecules of equivalent soluble fluorochrome (MESF), 44
Monoclonal antibodies, 4
  flow cytometry, 42
Monocytes, 46, 48
Mouse CTLL-2 cell line, 76
Mouth, 8
mRNA
  cytokines, 81
  growth factors, 89–90
Multiple myeloma, 10
Myasthenia gravis, 47
Myelocytes, 48
Myelodysplastic syndromes, 29–30
  5q-syndrome, 89
  FAB classification, 29–30
    stem cell transplantation, 10
Myeloperoxidase (MPO), 76, 157
  leukaemia diagnosis, 49
Myeloproliferative disorders, 30
  activation antigens, 58
  phenotypic analysis, 56

NADPH oxidase, 155–170
  activation, 162–165
  destructive roles, 167–168
  non-phagocytic systems, 166–167

oxygen sensing, 168–169
  plants, 167
NAP-2, 92, 98
  bioassays, 71
Natural killer (NK) cells, 46–47, 121, 125
Neuregulins, 92
Neurotrophin receptors, 97
Neutropenia, 9
  autoimmune, 57
N-nucleotides, 125
Nocardia spp., 165
Non-Hodgkin's lymphoma, 10, 54

Onco M, 74
Osteoarthritis, 167

p22-*phox*, 159–161, 165–166, 167
p40-*phox*, 161–162 , 165–166
p47-*phox*, 161–162, 165–166, 167
p67-*phox*, 161–162 , 165–166, 167
Pancytopenia, 6, 12
Paraformaldehyde, 43, 81
Paroxysmal nocturnal haemoglobinuria (PNH), 56
PDGF, 91
  receptor, 97
Pentose phosphate pathway, 156
Peripheral blood mononuclear cells (PBMCs), 45–47
Peripheral blood stem cell mobilization, 3, 57
Peroxynitrite, 157, 167
PF-4, 98
  bioassays, 71
Phagosomes, 158
Philadelphia chromosome
  acute lymphoblastic leukaemia, 20–21
  chronic myelocytic leukaemia, 26–27
Phosphatidylinositol-3-kinase (PI-3), 94
Phycoerythrin (PE), 43, 56
Plasmodium vivax, 98
Platelet peroxidase, 24
Pleiotropy, 89
Pneumococcus infections, 9
Pneumonitis, interstitial, 12
Polymerase chain reaction (PCR), 5, 52
Post-hypoxic polycythaemic mouse assay, 67

Prednisolone, 54
Proliferation bioassays, 76
Prolymphocytic leukaemia, 27, 55
Protein kinase C (PKC), 164
Pyrogen assay, 67

Quantum Red, 43

Radical derived products, 157
Radioimmunoassays (RIAs), 78–79
RANTES, 98
  bioassays, 71
  cell line-based assays, 75
Reactive oxygen species (ROS), 157,
    167–168
Receptor binding assays, 80
Receptor kinases, 91, 92, 95–98
Recombination activating gene (RAG)
    enzymes, 112–113, 125
Red-613, 43
Refractory anaemia (RA), 29
Refractory anaemia with excess blasts
    (RAEB), 10, 30
Refractory anaemia with excess blasts in
    transformation (RAEBt), 10, 30
Refractory anaemia with ring sideroblasts
    (RARS), 29–30
Renal disease, 150–151
Reporter gene-based assays, 78
Respiratory burst assays, 78
Respiratory burst phenomenon, 156
Retinoic acid receptor-alpha gene, 52
Reverse haemolytic plaque assay (RHPA),
    80–81
Reverse transcriptase-polymerase chain
    reaction (RT-PCR), 81
Rheumatoid arthritis, 167

Salmonella spp., 165
Saponin, 43, 81
Scatter factor, 97
Semliki Forest virus, 77
Sequence-specific oligonucleotide probes
    (SSOP), 5
Serpentine, 98
  receptors, 92
Serratia marcescens, 165

Sezary syndrome, 55
Skin, 7, 8
Splenic lymphoma with villous
    lymphocytes (SLVL), 27, 54
Splenomegaly, 6
src homology 2 (SH2), 94
src homology 3 (SH3) domains, 161
Staphylococcus infections, 8, 165
STAT family, 95
Stem cell factor (SCF), 91, 98–99, 106
  bioassays, 70
  cell line-based assays, 74
  functions, 88–89
  receptor, 97
  T cell development, 121
Stem cell transplantation, 1–16
  allogeneic, 2, 3–4
  autologous, 2, 3
  bone marrow harvest, 3
  complications, 7–8
  cord blood, 4, 13
  disease relapse, 11–12
  engraftment, 6
  ex vivo expansion, 13
  future prospects, 12–14
  gene therapy, 13–14
  graft engineering, 12–13
  graft failure, 6
  graft processing, 3–4
  graft versus host disease, 2, 4, 5, 7–8
  graft versus tumour effect, 11
  histocompatibility, 5
  history, 2–3
  immune reconstitution, 8
  immunology, 5
  indications, 10–11
  infection, 8–9, 14
  long-term complications, 9
  patient selection, 14
  peripheral blood stem cell (PBSC)
    mobilization, 3, 57
  preparative regimens, 5–6
  purging, 4–5
  rationale, 3
  secondary malignancies, 9
  sources of stem cells, 3–4
  syngeneic, 2

Stem cell transplantation, *contd.*
  umbilical cord blood, 4, 13
  unrelated donors, 13
Sudan Black B, 51
Superoxide dismutase (SOD), 157, 167
Suppressor T cells, 57

T cell leukaemia/lymphoma, 55
T cells, 5, 105, 118–132
  bone marrow, 121–123
  dual positive CD4+, CD8+ cells, 47
  extrathymic maturation, 131–132
  extra-thymic tolerance induction,
    130–131
  growth factors, 99–100
  helper:suppressor ratio, 57
  immune reconstitution, 8
  lineages, 123
  negative selection, 119, 120, 128–130
  positive selection, 118–119, 128–130
  progenitor cells, 121
  receptors, 123–130
  thymic development, 118–121, 125–130
Terminal deoxynucleotidyl transferase
    (TdT), 51, 53, 111, 117, 125
  leukaemia diagnosis, 49
  T cell ALL, 50
b-Thalassaemia, 14
Thiopurine, 22
Thrombocytopenia, 11
  autoimmune, 56
Thrombopoietin
  bioassays, 69
  cell line-based assays, 74, 76
  receptor, 93
Thymocytes, 99
Thymoma, 47
Thymus, 5
  B cells, 121
  microenvironment, 119–121
  stem cells, 121
  T cell deletion, 105
  T cell development, 118–121, 125–130
Thyroid tumours, 9
Thyroiditis, 47

Thyroxine, 9
Time of flight (TOF), 42
Total body irradiation, 6, 9
T-prolymphocytic leukaemia, 55
Transferrin receptor (CD71), 126
Transforming growth factor-beta, 64,
    91–92, 107
  cell line-based assays, 74
  reporter gene assay, 78
  sample preparation, 82
Trk receptors, 97
Tumour necrosis factor, 99, 107
  bioassays, 70
  family, 91
  receptor family, 98
  respiratory burst assays, 78
Tumour necrosis factor-alpha (TNF-
    alpha), 43, 66
  cell line-based assays, 75
  cell surface molecules, 76
  cytotoxic assays, 77
  immunoassays, 78
Tumour necrosis factor-beta (TNF-beta)
  cell line-based assays, 75
  cell surface molecules, 76
  cytotoxic assays, 77
  immunoassays, 78
Tyrosine kinase receptors, 91, 92, 95–98

Vaccination, 8
Vanishing bile duct syndrome, 7
Vascular endothelial growth factor
    receptors (VEGF-R), 97
VCAM-1, 106
Veno-occlusive disease, 12
Vesicular stomatitis virus, 77
Viral antigens, 43
VLA-4, 106

White blood cell count, 47
WHO International Standards, 82–84
  Reference Reagents, 83

Yeast artefactual chromosomes (YACs), 52,
    139